autism

PRESCHOOL ISSUES
IN AUTISM

CURRENT ISSUES IN AUTISM

Series Editors: Eric Schopler and Gary B. Mesibov

University of North Carolina School of Medicine
Chapel Hill, North Carolina

AUTISM IN ADOLESCENTS AND ADULTS
Edited by Eric Schopler and Gary B. Mesibov

BEHAVIORAL ISSUES IN AUTISM
Edited by Eric Schopler and Gary B. Mesibov

COMMUNICATION PROBLEMS IN AUTISM
Edited by Eric Schopler and Gary B. Mesibov

DIAGNOSIS AND ASSESSMENT IN AUTISM
Edited by Eric Schopler and Gary B. Mesibov

THE EFFECTS OF AUTISM ON THE FAMILY
Edited by Eric Schopler and Gary B. Mesibov

HIGH-FUNCTIONING INDIVIDUALS WITH AUTISM
Edited by Eric Schopler and Gary B. Mesibov

NEUROBIOLOGICAL ISSUES IN AUTISM
Edited by Eric Schopler and Gary B. Mesibov

PRESCHOOL ISSUES IN AUTISM
Edited by Eric Schopler, Mary E. Van Bourgondien,
  and Marie M. Bristol

SOCIAL BEHAVIOR IN AUTISM
Edited by Eric Schopler and Gary B. Mesibov

PRESCHOOL ISSUES IN AUTISM

Edited by

Eric Schopler,

Mary E. Van Bourgondien,

and

Marie M. Bristol

University of North Carolina School of Medicine
Chapel Hill, North Carolina

PLENUM PRESS • NEW YORK AND LONDON

Library of Congress Cataloging-in-Publication Data

Preschool issues in autism / edited by Eric Schopler, Mary E. Van
  Bourgondien, and Marie M. Bristol.
       p.   cm. -- (Current issues in autism)
    Includes bibliographical references and index.
    ISBN 0-306-44440-2
    1. Autism in children. 2. Autistic children. 3. Preschool
  children.   I. Schopler, Eric. II. Van Bourgondien, Mary Elizabeth.
  III. Bristol, Marie M. IV. Series.
    [DNLM: 1. Autism--in infancy & childhood--congresses. 2. Autism-
  -diagnosis--congresses. 3. Child Development--congresses. 4. Child
  Psychology--congresses. 5. Child, Preschool--congresses.   WM 203.5
  P928 1993]
  RJ506.A9P73   1993
  618.92'8982--dc20
  DNLM/DLC
  for Library of Congress   93-20597
                                                                    CIP

ISBN 0-306-44440-2

© 1993 Plenum Press, New York
A Division of Plenum Publishing Corporation
233 Spring Street, New York, N.Y. 10013

Printed in the United States of America

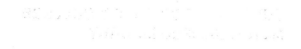

To young children with autism
and
the families who love and care for them,
with the hope that this volume will contribute
to earlier recognition of their strengths and their needs

Contributors

REBECCA ANGELL, Old Parish, Dungarvan, County Waterford, Ireland

MARIE M. BRISTOL, Division TEACCH, Department of Psychiatry, University of North Carolina at Chapel Hill, Chapel Hill, North Carolina 27599-7180

ROGER D. COX, Division TEACCH, Department of Psychiatry, University of North Carolina at Chapel Hill, Chapel Hill, North Carolina 27599-7180

CATHERINE LORD, Department of Psychiatry, University of Chicago, Chicago, Illinois 60637

LEE M. MARCUS, Division TEACCH, Department of Psychiatry, University of North Carolina at Chapel Hill, Chapel Hill, North Carolina 27599-7180

MARLENE MORELLI-ROBBINS, Department of Child and Family Studies, Florida Mental Health Institute, University of South Florida, Tampa, Florida 33612

J. GREGORY OLLEY, Clinical Center for the Study of Development and Learning, University of North Carolina at Chapel Hill, Chapel Hill, North Carolina 27599-7255

BARRY M. PRIZANT, Division of Communication Disorders, Emerson College, Boston, Massachusetts 02116

FRANK R. ROBBINS, Department of Child and Family Studies, Florida Mental Health Institute, University of South Florida, Tampa, Florida 33612

ERIC SCHOPLER, Division TEACCH, Department of Psychiatry, University of North Carolina at Chapel Hill, Chapel Hill, North Carolina 27599-7180

VICTORIA SHEA, Department of Psychiatry, University of North Carolina at Chapel Hill, Chapel Hill, North Carolina 27599-7180

WENDY L. STONE, Department of Pediatrics, Vanderbilt University School of Medicine, Nashville, Tennessee 37203

LAWRENCE T. TAFT, Division of Developmental Disabilities, University of Medicine and Dentistry of New Jersey, Robert Wood Johnson Medical School, New Brunswick, New Jersey 08903

JUDITH E. THIELE, Children's Rehabilitation Unit, University of Kansas Medical Center, Kansas City, Kansas 66160-7340

MARY E. VAN BOURGONDIEN, Division TEACCH, Department of Psychiatry, University of North Carolina at Chapel Hill, Chapel Hill, North Carolina 27599-7180

AMY M. WETHERBY, Department of Communication Disorders, Florida State University, Tallahassee, Florida 32306

Preface

In 1992, TEACCH, a division of the Department of Psychiatry at the University of North Carolina at Chapel Hill School of Medicine, celebrated its 20th anniversary as the first statewide, comprehensive service program for children and adults with autism. Since its inception, TEACCH has conducted over 6,000 evaluations, and it now serves more than 800 clients a year in its administrative center and its statewide network of six community-based regional centers. Through direct clinical services, consultation, teaching, and research, we at TEACCH have had the unique privilege of working with young children and their families since 1968, when TEACCH began as an NIMH research project. This volume is an attempt to draw on that experience and assess and share state-of-the-art techniques in early identification and services for young children with autism or related disorders.

This volume, like the other seven in the Current Issues in Autism series, grew from an annual conference. The book is not, however, simply a compilation of conference proceedings. Instead, selected conference participants were asked to develop chapters around the topics of their presentations. Other national or international experts in areas relevant to the conference theme were also asked to contribute chapters. The sum, then, presents an overview of some of the most current knowledge and best available practice.

Although aspects of identification of and service provision for young children with autism and related disorders have been touched upon in the other books in this series, recent advances in instrument development, efficacy research, and legal mandates for services make a volume devoted to young children particularly timely. The ambiguity of the diagnosis of autism in very young children has begun to yield to newly developed or modified instruments for diagnosis and assessment. Evidence of the efficacy of early and intensive intervention and the collaborative advocacy of parents and professionals have resulted in the passage, in the United States, of legislation that promises "free and appropriate" education and related services to children from birth. Set in that context, this volume synthesizes some of the most important theories, data, and clinical perspectives that will inform the best of those services. Although no single volume can include all that has been done in the burgeoning field of early intervention, we believe that the chapters in this volume will be useful in helping parents and professionals understand and implement state-of-the-art services for young children and their families.

ERIC SCHOPLER
MARY E. VAN BOURGONDIEN
MARIE M. BRISTOL

Acknowledgments

It is a pleasure to acknowledge the assistance of the many people who made this book a reality. First, we are indebted to Helen Garrison, who organized the conference that was the starting point for this book. As the audiences for these conferences have mushroomed, her creativity and organizational skills have been more than equal to the task. Thanks also to Ann Bashford, Jeanette Fergerson, and Vickie Weaver whose expert typing and secretarial assistance have been invaluable. Special thanks are due our TEACCH colleagues—clinical directors, therapists, teachers, and researchers—for stimulating ideas, constructive criticism, and the clinical reality check that informs all of our teaching, service, and research.

As with all our TEACCH efforts, this book would not be possible without the support of the Department of Psychiatry and the School of Medicine at the University of North Carolina at Chapel Hill. We are especially indebted to the North Carolina families who have shared with us their lives and their expertise. Finally, we thank the North Carolina State Legislature, whose continuing support for families and cost-effective services has been an inspiration for families everywhere.

Contents

Chapter 3

NORMAL CHILDHOOD DEVELOPMENT
FROM BIRTH TO FIVE YEARS

Roger D. Cox

Part II: Specific Aspects of Autism

Chapter 4

EARLY SOCIAL DEVELOPMENT IN AUTISM

Catherine Lord

Introduction and Overview

Introduction to Preschool Issues in Autism

MARIE M. BRISTOL and ERIC SCHOPLER

AN OLD AND NEW FRONTIER

This volume in the Plenum series, *Current Issues in Autism,* addresses the manifestations and treatment of autism and related disorders of communication and behavior in infants, toddlers, and preschool children with autism. As such, it has much in common with previous volumes while reflecting changes both in our understanding of autism and in society that make a focus on young children particularly compelling.

Although parents have long recognized symptoms later identified as autism in their infants or toddlers, professionals have been slow to agree on their significance. They have been slower still to decide on appropriate labels and treatments for those early symptoms. The impetus to provide early diagnosis and treatment for very young children with autism has been provided by a transformation in our understanding of the role of parents in this disorder, an evolution in the definition of autism, an emerging consensus regarding the efficacy of early intervention, and federal legislation mandating services for this age group. Serving these young children is complicated, in turn, by the normal

MARIE M. BRISTOL and ERIC SCHOPLER • Division TEACCH, Department of Psychiatry, University of North Carolina at Chapel Hill, Chapel Hill, North Carolina 27599-7180.

Preschool Issues in Autism, edited by Eric Schopler *et al.* Plenum Press, New York, 1993.

variation in early development and the ambiguity of differential diagnosis and prognosis at this young age.

ROLE OF PARENTS IN AUTISM

The changed role of parents has provided a major impetus for early diagnosis and treatment of autism. Kanner (1943) originally defined autism as an inborn defect, but this explanation was soon overshadowed by the prevailing psychoanalytic zeitgeist which saw the child's problems as a reflection of rejecting or defective parenting. Both a failure of empirical research to substantiate any such parenting cause (Cantwell & Baker, 1984; Schopler, in press) and the increasing evidence of a biological basis for autism (Schopler & Mesibov, 1987) have led to a reconceptualization of the parent's role in autism (Bristol & Schopler, 1989).

Initially scapegoated (Schopler, Brehm, Kinsbourne, & Reichler, 1971) for their child's disorder and even remanded to treatment that sought to change their character or personality, parents are now seen as cotherapists in the treatment of their child (Lord, Bristol, & Schopler, this volume; Schopler, Mesibov, Shigley, & Bashford, 1984) and as vocal and effective advocates for early and appropriate treatment. Freed from the onus of unwarranted blame for their child's disorder, parents, aided by informed professionals, have insisted instead on the validity of their early observations of their own child's development (Schopler & Reichler, 1972). They also have recognized both the need for and the value of early treatment when signs and symptoms cause concern. Recently (Bristol & Schopler, 1989), the American Psychiatric Association officially recognized this changed role for parents in the etiology and treatment of autism, and in so doing, implicitly endorsed the necessity of responding to parents' requests for early diagnosis and intervention.

EVOLUTION IN THE DEFINITION OF AUTISM

Changes in the definition of autism also favor a focus on earlier diagnosis and treatment (Schopler, 1983; Rutter & Schopler, 1978, 1988). Since Kanner first defined the autism syndrome in 1943, criteria for diagnosis of autism have been among the more consistent in the lexicon of psychiatry. However, based on extensive empirical research, there have been refinements in the definition that favor earlier diagnosis and treatment. Although it is clear that some cases of autism do not develop until 36 months of age, research has substantiated that most cases can be recognized, at least in retrospect, by 2 years of age (Short & Schopler, 1988; Volkmar & Cohen, 1988).

Problems of socialization and communication have always been considered the hallmarks of autism. However, recent research has demonstrated that it is not the *lack* of either language or socialization that discriminates autism from mental retardation or other disorders, but rather a difference in the quality and use of communication and socialization, particularly in the initiation and reciprocity of interaction. This is a subtle but important refinement in our understanding of autism reflected in current diagnostic criteria in the *Diagnostic and Statistical Manual* (American Psychiatric Association, 1987). It means that it is no longer necessary to wait until age 5 or 6 to see if the child develops language with characteristic reversal of pronouns and echolalic features or to see if the child will develop sophisticated social interactions at school age. Increasing attention can be given, for example, to whether toddlers communicate, verbally or nonverbally, to meet their needs, and more important, whether they initiate and sustain interaction with another person through eye contact, gestures, or other nonverbal means.

A growing recognition of the interactive functions served by unusual vocal or other behaviors has also given us new insights into preverbal communication and what were once seen only as disruptive or bizarre behaviors. Focusing on communication instead of language and on initiation and reciprocity of interaction instead of social skills alone allows us to begin diagnosis and treatment earlier in the child's development.

CONSENSUS ON EFFICACY OF EARLY INTERVENTION

Findings from a variety of early intervention programs (Olley, Robbins, & Morelli-Robbins, this volume) indicate that young children with autism do not outgrow their symptoms without treatment and that those who do receive early and intensive intervention make significant and often dramatic improvement. Although all the data do not yet demonstrate which specific features are critical to early intervention success, the evidence that early intervention is effective in improving the lives of both children and their families continues to accumulate. This has been one of the incentives for producing this book. In its chapters, the authors share their knowledge about the earliest manifestations of this disorder and its treatment. Data suggesting dramatic improvements with intensive intervention for the most mildly impaired preschool children also heighten the urgency of identifying especially those children whose parents would have been counseled previously "to wait and see if he outgrows it."

PUBLIC LAW 99-457

In 1986 the US Congress passed legislation now known as Public Law 99-457 (Thiele, this volume). To continue to receive federal preschool special education funds, states must provide free multidisciplinary diagnosis, assessment, and appropriate public education to all 3- to 5-year-old handicapped children while extending to their parents essentially the same due process rights previously guaranteed to school-aged children. The legislation also provides incentives to serve infants and toddlers from birth through age 2, and encourages extensive early identification and treatment. Since eligibility for services and funding hinges on meeting federal or state criteria for disability or risk, this legislation provides a strong impetus to establish criteria for early diagnosis and to clarify what "appropriate" education and related services should be.

OVERVIEW

This volume addresses aspects of autism in young children seen from the perspective of normal child and family development. It includes issues of diagnosis, assessment, and treatment—global and specific, theoretical and programmatic, practical and legal. It is written primarily for practitioners and policymakers in the field and, as such, focuses on key concepts in each area rather than on an exhaustive review of all pertinent research.

Introduction and Overview

Part I, Introduction and Overview, introduces autism as seen from the perspective of normal family life and child development. The book begins with a parent's discussion of autism, not in the context of theory or research, but in the context of a normal family with solicitous, well-meaning relatives and friends, siblings, support groups, and daily tensions. In Chapter 2, Angell describes the gradual and painful discovery of autism in her son, the prodigy who hummed symphonies at the age of 17 months. She takes the reader on the roundabout path she followed from her beautiful child's uneventful birth through vague uneasiness about his failure to communicate, on through diagnosis and advocacy for services as the family moved from Ireland, to North Carolina, and back to Ireland again.

This chapter is different from others published by parents of older children looking back on this early period from the healing distance of a decade or more. The pain this mother feels is poignantly captured in excerpts from her journal entries as doubt graduates to worry and the quest for confirming diagnosis and appropriate services begins. Angell captures well both the unique bond she shares with other mothers of children like her own and the need to set boundaries on activities on behalf of her autistic child in order to preserve some normalcy for herself and the rest of her family. She concludes with advice to other parents and a frank and touching account of the tension and ambivalence that these children bring to their families.

As Angell points out, it is only in grasping both the range and the limits of what is normal that the presence and severity of the disorder can be recognized in very young children. This focus, autism as seen in the context of normal development, is the topic of Chapter 3. In it, Cox presents an admirable review of normal aspects of development during the first 5 years of life. He focuses on those that involve moving toward, communicating, and socializing with others. He begins with a discussion of motor development, usually the area of greatest strength for young children with autism. He ends that discussion with the cautionary note that even well-developed motor skills do not ensure that the child with autism will develop the sense of danger or cautiousness that protects most nonhandicapped children from the consequences of their actions. Illustrating his points with a discussion of types and uses of toys, Cox then details the development of cognitive ability from earliest infancy through the use of symbolic and abstract thought. This progression and the divergences from normal development in autism are particularly clear in his discussion of social-emotional development in infants and the emergence of imitation and response to human faces and voices. He points out that most of these social-affective goals are largely achieved in nonhandicapped infants in their first months of life. This chapter highlights the severity of the communicative and social-affective deficits seen in children with autism when compared with their nonhandicapped peers.

Specific Aspects of Autism

Each of the three chapters of Part II, Specific Aspects of Autism, is an in-depth discussion of one particular aspect of autism. In discussing competence in complex skills during the preschool period, it is clear that no single domain of development is adequate to explain success or failure. Most skills of concern in very young children with autism involve the coordination of at least cognitive, social, and communicative components. Even teaching such a seemingly straightforward skill as riding a tricycle is influenced not only by the motor development necessary to push the pedals, but by the cognitive and communicative development and social motivation required to understand the instructions, to imitate and ride with other children, to perceive the function of the bike as a means of transportation (rather than focusing on a wheel or a pattern of shining spokes), and to have the social judgment needed not to ride the tricycle into the street. However, to simplify presentation, we asked each author in this section to focus on one particular aspect of early development in autism, knowing full well, as we now caution our readers, that this division into different aspects of development is for clarity of exposition only.

The first of these chapters, Chapter 4, by Lord, addresses early social development, arguably the most persistent and handicapping aspect of autism. Lord offers a thorough discussion of four social behavior categories: sociability, attachments, understanding and expressing emotions, and behaviors related to social success. She first reviews the research on social behaviors in each category that discriminate young children with autism from mental-age-matched peers and then discusses strategies and problems in assessing these social deficits. This includes a description of two instruments developed recently: the Autism Diagnostic Interview (Le Couteur *et al.*, 1989) and the Autism Diagnostic Observation Schedule (Lord *et al.*, 1989) that show promise in diagnosing and assessing social and communicative behavior of children with verbal mental ages of 3 years and up.

Going beyond a discussion of standardized assessment instruments, Lord focuses on the identification of behaviors specific to autism including methods for determining them. She provides insights into separating children's responses to structure and routine from spontaneous social behaviors, including a discussion of the differing roles that mothers, fathers, and therapists can play in assessing different kinds of social behaviors. The final section of this chapter outlines goals for social interventions with young autistic children and includes seven principles for providing treatment of social deficits in young children with autism.

In Chapter 5, Prizant and Weatherby discuss communication that is central to diagnosis, assessment, and treatment efforts with preschool children. The chapter is written with a special emphasis on developmental and pragmatic approaches to assessment and intervention. It also includes the role of family and caregivers as partners in helping children develop communication and social-affective competence. The chapter is significant for its thoughtful melding of both developmental and functional approaches to assessment and intervention. Prizant and Weatherby provide guidelines for both contexts and content of communicative assessment, including four questions to be used to assign communicative level, and guidelines for establishing priorities and procedures for communicative intervention. In forming priorities and procedures for communicative enhancement, they consider the following goals: to expand the child's repertoire of communicative functions; to help the child develop more sophisticated and effective means of communicating (including ways to repair communicative breakdowns and improve the readability and social acceptability of the child's communication); and to enhance the reciprocity of the child's communication. The chapter contains helpful indicators or contraindicators for the use of augmentative or nonspeech systems. It concludes with a discussion of the role of structure in enhancing communicative competence.

Behavior problems in preschool children are the topic of Chapter 6. Van Bourgondien reviews some of the behavior problems seen most frequently in preschool children with autism and relates them both to problems in normal development and to underlying deficits in autism. Using the TEACCH iceberg metaphor, Van Bourgondien demonstrates how typical autism problems such as rigid food preferences or eating inedible substances may be reflections of underlying deficits such as impaired taste perception or insistence on sameness rather than deliberately oppositional behavior. Van Bourgondien describes a six-step problem solving approach for working with parents and teachers to develop an intervention program to change either the child's behavior or the attitudes and environments in which the problem behaviors occur.

Diagnostic, Assessment, and Programmatic Aspects

The final section, Part III, Diagnostic, Assessment, and Programmatic Aspects, covers the more global aspects of good practice. These begin with overall diagnosis and assessment, both psychoeducational and medical, and interpreting the diagnosis to parents. Current best practice in programmatic intervention is presented, first with a description of a single program, then with a look at factors related to successful outcome across programs, and finally with a discussion of the federal legislation that has spawned much of the current interest in serving toddlers and preschoolers with autism.

In Chapter 7, Marcus and Stone discuss diagnosis and assessment in the young child with autism as a crucial first step in developing and planning comprehensive treatment and education programs. They review empirical data on social, communicative, and repetitive or restrictive behaviors that differentiate young children with autism from nonhandicapped children or children with other disorders. This chapter is significant for its discussion of both the empirical support found for characteristics such as imitation previously thought to differentiate autism from other disorders. It also covers other characteristics such as the presumed pervasive lack of affection and attachment, which have not had sustained empirical support as discriminators of autism. Marcus and Stone also point out gaps in our present knowledge of development, particularly of social and repetitive behaviors in young children with normal development or with developmental disorders. Clinicians will find in this chapter helpful discussions of problems in diagnosing and assessing young children as well as information and management strategies to overcome those formidable obstacles.

Autism is increasingly recognized as a biologically based disorder. Although many questions remain regarding etiology, particularly in specific cases, a comprehensive diagnosis and assessment also includes consideration of medical disorders that cause, occur with, or may be mistaken for autism. In Chapter 8, Taft reviews a number of these developmental disorders of the central nervous system that have been associated frequently with autism. Some, such as phenylketonuria, are treatable and reversible conditions. Taft provides helpful guidelines for differentiating this and other disorders, such as Rett syndrome, which have a different prognosis and treatment from autism. Knowledge of the disorders described in this chapter will be invaluable both for differential diagnosis and for helping clinicians make decisions regarding referral for genetic counseling.

In Chapter 9, Shea outlines ways in which the interpretive conference with parents can be used to convey and clarify the diagnostic and assessment information found, to assist parents with their emotional reactions to this information, and to make concrete plans to provide for both the child's and the family's needs. In clear and straightforward language, she discusses the goals and content of the interpretive session, principles for professional conduct in this situation, and special issues related to diagnosis and prognosis for preschool children. Shea clearly places the interpretive conference in the context of building a respectful, supportive, and collaborative relationship with parents, and to minimize their confusion and pain. Shea points out that interpretation requires preparation, skill, and honesty on the part of professionals in order to avoid what parents too often report as one of the most devastating experiences of their lives.

The first three chapters of Part III address specific facets of intervention—social, communicative, or behavioral. Chapter 10 describes how selected aspects of assessment and intervention are brought together in TEACCH preschool classrooms. Division TEACCH (*T*reatment and *E*ducation of *A*utistic and related *C*ommunication handicapped *CH*ildren) is North Carolina's statewide program for children with autism or related communication handicaps and their families. In this chapter, Lord, Bristol, and Schopler describe the TEACCH family-focused program of early intervention which has both center-based and home-based components. After discussing the differences both between preschool and older children with autism and between preschool children with autism and children with other disorders on issues of diagnosis, assessment, family situations, and other relevant issues, the TEACCH preschool program is presented in light of all of these issues.

The authors describe the role of parents and teachers in assessment and intervention and the collaborative development of programming aimed especially at increasing spontaneous communication and socialization. The focus of the chapter is on the use of structured teaching in preventing or reducing behavior problems, increasing independence, and reducing both child and teacher stress. This highly individualized program uses the child's visual and spatial strengths to compensate for social and communication deficits through the physical arrangement of the classroom, visual systems for schedules and transitions, individualized work systems, and task and material structure. The authors conclude with a discussion of the concept of a continuum of services as more than the provision of services provided by TEACCH over time. TEACCH offers a continuum of service approaches and sites for the same age group and a continuum of options for the coordination of these services within the community.

In Chapter 11, Olley and his associates review a number of current preschool programs in light of factors reported to be related to effective early intervention in autism. The authors briefly describe 10 of the best known programs for preschool children with autism and then evaluate curriculum or program characteristics, measurement, and dissemination practices of these exemplary programs. All of these programs include components found by Simeonsson, Olley, and Rosenthal (1987) to be related to effective early intervention. These involve a behavior orientation, parent involvement, initiation of treatment at an early age, relatively intensive services, and a specific focus on generalization. Although the programs differ in many ways, Olley and his associates conclude that they have many things in common. These include the consistent and systematic application of teaching methods, the teaching of social competence and communication in a social context as a means to prevent or reduce behavior problems, an individualized approach to parent involvement, collection of multiple dependent measures of outcome including assessment of social validity or meaningfulness of program gains, and efforts at dissemination and replication. The authors also describe gaps in our knowledge of *what* has worked for *whom*.

They discuss the continuing questions of optimum age for beginning intervention and optimum intensity necessary for good outcome. The authors point out that these programs serve children with a range of abilities. Some but not all serve children with neurological or other complications likely to affect outcome. In describing the variety of settings in which these programs are conducted, it is clear that setting alone is not the major determinant of good or poor outcome. The authors conclude with a list of questions which they expect to be answered in the next decade of research.

Finally, in Chapter 12, Thiele describes Public Law 99–457, which provides strong exhortation with nominal resources for states to provide services for children from birth to 5 years, including toddlers and children who have or are at risk for autism. Thiele briefly reviews the major provisions of that remarkable piece of legislation which made a major commitment to our youngest and most vulnerable children at a time of unprecedented budget cuts and restrictions in social services.

CONCLUSIONS

The chapters in this volume make a strong case for early identification and treatment of children with autism. It appears that autism can be diagnosed in very young children using the triad of social, communicative, and repetitive or restricted activities or interests specified in the current definition, even though both diagnosis and prognosis is more ambiguous at this age than later. Clearly the form that these symptoms take in very young children differs from that in older children or adults. More empirical work is needed to separate assumption from fact in early diagnostic criteria, especially in the area of repetitive and restricted behaviors and interests.

However, this volume reports on an emerging consensus that although it is difficult to definitively establish the diagnosis of autism in toddlers and preschool children, early intervention is important in facilitating learning and in preventing the development of secondary behavior problems caused by the frustration of being unable to communicate and relate to others. Initial data suggest that "earlier" is, in fact, better and may have dramatic results, especially for mildly impaired children. Across all chapters there is a consensus that effective programs include high degrees of parental involvement, structure, ongoing assessment, and individualized programming adapted to the child's uneven developmental levels across skill areas. In autism this is best accomplished by building on visual and spatial strengths and focusing on spontaneous initiation instead of just compliance. Effective interventions appear to be relatively intensive, intrusive, and interactional, requiring adaptations from both the child and others in the child's environment. There is no evidence in these chapters or known to the editors that merely placing children with autism in classes with nonhandicapped children or children with other disabilities will enable them to develop spontaneous communication and social interaction.

Exciting research is currently underway to examine issues of medical etiology, diagnosis, assessment, and treatment of young children. Among other studies at Division TEACCH, research is presently in progress to identify indices of autism in children under three, and to perfect a multiaxial system of classifying autism which should have important implications for both intervention and prediction with this age group. Pilot work is also underway to identify inherited patterns of language, learning, and social deficits that might ultimately point to a genetic contribution in a subset of young children with autism. Although there are still far too many unanswered questions about this young age group, we trust that this book contributes by reviewing the current state-of-the-art in the continuing search for answers.

REFERENCES

American Psychiatric Association. (1987). *Diagnostic and statistical manual of mental disorders* (3rd ed., rev.). Washington, DC: Author.

Bristol, M., & Schopler, E. (1989). The family in the treatment of autism. In American Psychiatric Association, *Treatments of psychiatric disorders: A task force report of the American Psychiatric Association* (pp. 249–266). Washington, DC: American Psychiatric Association.

Cantwell, D., & Baker, L. (1984). Research concerning families of children with autism. In E. Schopler & G. Mesibov (Eds.), *The effects of autism on the family* (pp. 41–63). New York: Plenum.

Kanner, L. (1943). Autistic disturbances of affective contact. *Nervous Child, 2,* 217–250.

Le Couteur, A., Rutter, M., Lord, C., Rios, P., Robertson, S., Holdgrafer, M., & McLennan, J. (1989). Autism diagnostic interview: A standardized investigator-based instrument. *Journal of Autism and Developmental Disorders, 19,* 363–387.

Lord, C., Rutter, M., Goode, S., Heemsbergen, J., Jordan, H., Mawhood, L., & Schopler, E. (1989). Autism diagnostic observation schedule: A standardized observation of communicative and social behavior. *Journal of Autism and Developmental Disorders, 19,* 185–212.

Rutter, M., & Schopler, E. (Eds.). (1978). *Autism: A reappraisal of concepts and treatment.* New York: Plenum.

Rutter, M., & Schopler, E. (1988). Autism and pervasive developmental disorders: Concepts and diagnostic issues. In E. Schopler & G. Mesibov (Eds.), *Diagnosis and assessment in autism* (pp. 15–36). New York: Plenum.

Schopler, E. (in press). Neurobiologic correlates in the classification and study of autism. In S. Broman & J. Grafman (Eds.), *Atypical cognitive deficits in developmental disorders: Implication for brain function*. Hillsdale, NJ: Erlbaum.

Schopler, E. (1983). New developments in the definition and diagnosis of autism. In B. Lahey & A. Kazdin (Eds.), *Advances in clinical child psychology, Vol. 6* (pp. 93–127). New York: Plenum.

Schopler, E., Brehm, S., Kinsbourne, M., & Reichler, R. (1971). Effects of treatment structure on development in autistic children. *Archives of General Psychiatry, 24,* 415–421.

Schopler, E., & Mesibov, G. (Eds.). (1987). *Neurobiological issues in autism.* New York: Plenum.

Schopler, E., Mesibov, G., Shigley, R., & Bashford, A. (1984). Helping autistic children through their parents: The TEACCH model. In E. Schopler & G. Mesibov (Eds.), *The effects of autism on the family* (pp. 65–81). New York: Plenum.

Schopler, E., & Reichler, R. (1972). How well do parents understand their own psychotic child? *Journal of Autism and Childhood Schizophrenia, 2,* 387–400.

Short, A., & Schopler, E. (1988). Factors relating to age of onset in autism. *Journal of Autism and Developmental Disorders, 18,* 207–216.

Simeonsson, R., Olley, J., & Rosenthal, S. (1987). Early intervention for children with autism. In M. Guralnick & F. Bennett (Eds.), *The effectiveness of early intervention for at-risk and handicapped children* (pp. 275–296). New York: Academic.

Volkmar, F., & Cohen, D. (1988). Classification and diagnosis of childhood autism. In E. Schopler & G. Mesibov (Eds.), *Diagnosis and assessment in autism* (pp. 71–89). New York: Plenum.

2

A Parent's Perspective on the Preschool Years

REBECCA ANGELL

He hummed symphonies at the tender age of 17 months. By 20 months he had invented his first original melody. A favorite pastime consisted of studying two storybooks at a time, searching for words such as *tales* or *fairy* that might appear in both.

Although our son displayed these obvious signs of intelligence, we sometimes wondered why he had never said a single word—not *mama* or *ball* or *dog*—nothing. Eoin (pronounced like the Welsh *Owen*) made all sorts of charming baby noises, but even the fondest parent would not have interpreted them as words.

He displayed no interest in walking or even crawling at 12 to 14 months, when his peers were toddling about. "He's just too busy composing," we told our friends. Our uneasiness was tinged with pride at his unusual accomplishments.

As Eoin grew older, we were increasingly puzzled by his behavior, but it did not seem typical of any particular abnormality. When he was 3 years and 10 months old our backward prodigy was officially diagnosed as mildly autistic. The path to this label was gradual and roundabout.

REBECCA ANGELL • Old Parish, Dungarvan, County Waterford, Ireland.

Preschool Issues in Autism, edited by Eric Schopler *et al.* Plenum Press, New York, 1993.

DISCOVERY AND DIAGNOSIS

His First Year

Eoin was born on a sunny May day in Waterford, Ireland. His name is the ancient Irish Gaelic equivalent of John, meaning gracious gift of God. Eoin's birth was unmedicated and fairly uneventful. He weighed 8 pounds and 14 ounces, performed all of the functions expected of newborns, and went home from the hospital the next day.

He was a beautiful baby. Articles claiming that most autistic children are beautiful inspire me to scoff at such illogic and recall the homely autistic children I know. Nonetheless, I became so used to comments on his beauty that I noticed only the occasional instances when people failed to comment on it, rather than the numerous times they did.

We thought Eoin was normal. He enjoyed being held and was generally contented, a "good baby," in Irish parlance. Was he too "good," too placid? It is difficult to judge in retrospect, but I do not think so.

Some autistic children develop normally until around age 2, when they regress, withdraw, and begin to exhibit autistic characteristics. Eoin did not do this. Although we did not perceive it at the time, his behavior gradually began to deviate from the norm during his first year.

I clearly remember my first misgivings, after we had moved from Ireland back to North Carolina. I was sitting on the floor beside our 10-month-old son while skimming through a friend's book that outlined a baby's first year month by month. Uneasily, I noted that Eoin was doing some things that were beyond the 12-month level, yet he was on the 2- and 3-month levels in several areas. Despite the book's disclaimer that not all babies could be expected to progress exactly as outlined, it did seem peculiar that Eoin's development followed these standards so erratically.

My husband and I disliked the current "super baby" theories. We were determined to stimulate and encourage our child, but not push him. We prided ourselves on not wanting to force our progeny into any standardized molds. I dismissed the book as being too rigid, but could not erase my doubts. Over the next few years I was torn between scorning this type of book and permitting myself a few anxiety-laden peeks.

John and I did not realize our inexperience as parents would prove a handicap. We were middle-class, college-educated Americans. In our 7 years of marriage we had traveled widely, worked hard, and were now eager to be parents. I was 29; John was 30. We had learned about natural childbirth and read the standard childrearing books but were naive about normal development. Although many of a baby's actions and characteristics cannot be quantified, an experienced eye might have perceived that something was seriously wrong before we did.

I am not sure why I began keeping a detailed journal of Eoin's development; perhaps I did so because I am an inveterate notetaker, or because I was excited about becoming a parent. As months passed, I gradually suspected that Eoin was somehow different; I wanted to record those differences on paper.

His Second Year

Eoin was 13 months old when I first compared his actions to another child's and felt troubled. Another couple and their 8-month-old daughter came to our apartment for dinner. Although this child was 5 months younger than Eoin, I noticed that she was much more agile and able to feed herself. In my journal I noted, "She is more independent, willing to be without Mommy. By catering to Eoin all the time, I suppose we made him clingy."

We became expert at rationalizing in these early years. Eoin's lack of physical accomplishments could easily be explained because he was chubby, unlikely to compete with a wiry child. Eoin was content to stay planted in one spot, although he occasionally rolled partway across the room. Gradually he learned to creep and first crawled at nearly 15 months. This seemed peculiar, yet we were pleased that during this period he became adept at pushing geometrical shapes through the proper slots in a toy mailbox and spent considerable time devising different combinations for a set of stacking blocks. His ability to work puzzles far outstripped his mobility.

By the time Eoin was 17 months old we were accustomed to shrugging off inquiries about whether he was walking yet. After all, a normal, intelligent friend assured us that he had not taken his first step until after he turned 2. In addition, it seemed that Eoin's sedentary state was partially compensated for by the emergence of unusual musical abilities.

John's mother, a violinist, asked to hear our tape of a virtuoso solo, Maurice Ravel's "Tsigane." Later that day we heard 17-month-old Eoin humming the melody perfectly, adroitly switching from major to minor key. In the next few months Eoin's hummed repertoire blossomed to about 45 pieces, reflecting our interest in classical music. Despite this musical interest, Eoin refused even to listen to children's songs. Years later we realized that he disliked songs with words because he did not understand them.

We knew Eoin would walk someday; he finally did on the day he turned 18 months old. At his 18-month checkup, the pediatrician pronounced him in excellent health, in or above the 100th percentile for size. I was a bit irritated that the overly talkative nurse made disparaging comments about things Eoin should be doing, but the doctor seemed to consider him a fine specimen. Perhaps he might have been more critical had he not been a friend of John's parents and served as John's pediatrician, as well.

My husband and I love music. At first we shared this interest with Eoin by playing tapes. Soon we cautiously began taking him to concerts. Although some members of the audience watched disapprovingly as he crawled into his seat, they soon forgot about him as he quietly listened to the music. At 19 months, he was thrilled by a live performance of Tchaikovsky's ballet, "The Nutcracker."

Given this stimulation, we were not surprised when, at 20 months, Eoin passed another peculiar milestone by inventing his first melody. Since one of us was always with Eoin and was thus aware of what he was hearing, we knew the melody was original. Eoin followed with four other "compositions" over the next 2 years before the composing ceased.

Also at 20 months, Eoin was interested in letters and words. He scrutinized his alphabet blocks and grouped them by letter. He buttonholed us to point out a word that he found in two books, tediously pointing back and forth, back and forth, as if to make sure we truly comprehended. My journal entry was partially prophetic: "It's hard to believe that anyone so interested in this sort of thing won't be reading for several years! Maybe he'll read before he talks!"

His failure to talk was baffling. "Bye" was Eoin's only word at 22 months. I wondered why he never attempted *mama* or *dada,* but he obviously loved us and was strongly attached to us. "Any words yet?" became the routine greeting from a friend whose talkative son was Eoin's age. Eventually she stopped asking.

Other friends readily provided reassurance. After all, didn't Einstein take his time learning to talk? My mother said I had been very slow to talk until I turned 2, when I jumped from using a few words to speaking in sentences in the space of a few weeks. It was easy to dredge up cases of brilliant late bloomers.

"He's probably understanding every word," people said consolingly. Of course, we wanted to believe that; we did not realize how little he comprehended.

It is difficult for people to be objective about their own children, particularly when a child diverges from the mainstream. As Eoin approached 2, my journal became peppered by negativism and doubt: "Eoin was late to crawl, late to walk, late to feed himself, late to toilet train—is this due to some quirk of his, or because we haven't pushed him, or what?"

His Third Year

The word "independence" began to appear with increasing frequency in my journal. I commented on the trait when I observed it, but wondered why Eoin exhibited it so seldom. Although Eoin had a hearty appetite, he absolutely refused to try to feed himself with a determination that seemed stronger than a child's normal obstinacy. He was 3 years and 1 week old when he finally picked up his spoon and fork.

The birth of Eoin's sister, Lia, when Eoin was 29 months old gave us further opportunity to rationalize: after all, many older siblings regress to compete with a new baby.

When does doubt graduate to worry? I did not admit this gradual progression even to my husband, and only rarely to myself.

Just after Eoin turned 3, John entered seminary in a small North Carolina town. I took the children to the free local health center there for vaccinations and checkups. Many of the children at the center obviously were deprived emotionally and intellectually, as well as economically. Yet even these children who received attention primarily in the form of slaps or curses seemed superior to our child, who was surrounded by love and attention. I morosely watched Eoin fix his attention on a stuffed animal while other youngsters arranged the chairs like a jungle gym and chattered effortlessly.

I have never been confident. Despite the patent illogic in my thinking, I sometimes tormented myself by wondering how I could be such a defective parent that I could rear a child who did not even approximate the norm, yet did not seem to have any malady that could be identified and treated.

I do not know whether Eoin gradually became more withdrawn or whether he was just approaching an age where increasing interaction was expected, yet did not appear.

I flip through photograph albums to examine his first years. His attention was engaged, his expression lively, his contact direct. Who could find fault with this bright-eyed, laughing child in the pictures? Then I recall a conflicting image of Eoin sitting at his grandparents' dinner table on many occasions, gazing out the window at the graceful trees in the backyard. At the time his reverie seemed charmingly pensive; we did not think of withdrawal at the time.

Soon after Eoin was 3, I unwittingly became the first to make the correct diagnosis: "It is frustrating that he often seems to ignore people, won't answer questions, lives in his own world, won't listen to stories, has definite, fixed ideas, always takes the same walk. Is he similar, in a way, to those kids who can't be reached?" I vaguely recalled the term autism from a college psychology course, but I knew our son did not resemble the textbook photograph of a boy who withdrew into a fetal position. I dismissed the possibility of autism until Eoin's evaluators mentioned it nearly a year later.

Eoin's increasing rigidity was a problem, but it did not seem major. If plans were changed hastily, or rigid routines were not followed, Eoin's affability abruptly switched to anxiety, accompanied by what seemed like incredible stubbornness. Occasionally he had tantrums, but we considered those normal. Eoin trained me to follow certain procedures in a specific order. We learned to avoid activities or places that might trigger a tantrum or activate his phobias of dogs and gray-haired people.

Some of Eoin's activities that we later recognized as autistic seemed odd or even amusing. We marveled at his sense of order when he lined up toy animals or little cars and trucks in long, perfect rows.

For a few weeks he was fascinated with shoes. Eoin raided all of our closets to produce a serpentine column of shoes and books, marching from room to room.

We appreciated his orderliness. It seemed nice to have a child who put things back in their places. Occasionally, Eoin chose an unusual resting spot for an object. He decided that a tiny toy excavator should sit on top of the living room bookcase rather than be relegated to the car and truck box. The toys' whereabouts did not really matter to me, but the game was intriguing: I would return the excavator to its box; it inevitably reappeared on the bookcase. I never saw Eoin move it.

Eoin was unusually obedient in these early years. If told not to touch something, he didn't, period. He did not exhibit the balkiness and contrariness characteristic of a 2-year-old until he was 7.

Despite Eoin's inability to do many things, new abilities arose. His tactile hypersensitivity made opening a door or grasping a pencil difficult, yet we discovered that his fine motor skills requiring a light touch were unusually good. We bought a set of miniature wooden farm and zoo animals, some as tiny as half an inch high. Eoin devised many different arrangements. He positioned animals in stacks that seemed impossibly precarious but did not tumble down. We never equaled his feat of balancing seven pink pigs on each other's curved backs.

Eoin's difficulty in gripping a pencil or crayon limited him to producing scribbles. He fared better grasping a paintbrush. Framed watercolors grace the living rooms of both sets of grandparents. Both paintings are abstract, but unusually beautiful. I watched him slowly and systematically paint both, obviously following a plan known only to him.

As Eoin grew older, we realized that his memory was unusually good. When he was 31 months old, he led me on a walk past 10 identical brick buildings and flights of stairs, to the door of an apartment we had moved from 16 months earlier. Between the ages of 3 and 4, he showed on numerous occasions that he recognized people he had not seen since he was less than 2.

Eoin's expressive vocabulary consisted of only four words by the time he was 33 months old. Yet when we drove along a busy strip of fast food restaurants several months later, he said what clearly sounded like an Irish word: *bó*, which means *cow*. I scanned the pizza parlors and hamburger joints and finally saw a large plaster holstein perched on the roof of a dairy bar. The word lay, unused, in Eoin's memory for nearly 2 years. Later he began interjecting about a dozen Irish words into his English vocabulary. Naturally this did not help people understand this child whose articulation was fuzzy and sentence structure primitive.

Because he could become totally absorbed in one activity or emotion, Eoin sometimes displayed a rare joy that seemed like total happiness untainted by other feelings. This was particularly evident at the beach, where Eoin would dash into the water and stay as long as we permitted. He displayed no interest in sand or shells, just sheer exultation at being in the rough waves that occasionally bowled him over but did not lessen his enthusiasm.

THE DIAGNOSTIC PROCESS

The first official warning that something was wrong was at a routine doctor's checkup at the local health center during the August after Eoin turned 3. Physically, he was fine. However, the pediatrician commented that we should visit a psychologist to see why Eoin was not talking more. As I rattled off his accomplishments, she gently commented that even if he were a genius, he would have to communicate better. She referred us to the Developmental Evaluation Clinic, a state agency serving children from birth to age 9.

The 2-month wait for that appointment dragged by slowly. When we saw the psychologist, she administered the blocks and picture games that soon became routine. Then we talked. I sensed that behind her liberal sprinkling of psychological jargon, she was as baffled as we were. My notes record: "Oral motor problem? Large motor problem? Balance? Do some physical problems make him react emotionally and shut things out (I doubt it)? . . . She questions his cognitive emotional abilities and wonders about 'socio-emotional' growth."

In contrast, her conclusion was unscientific: "You can just look at his eyes and see that he is bright." She suggested that Eoin be given a full evaluation by the clinic's staff. Meanwhile, she advised us to read about specific learning disabilities. I must have seemed too cavalier about Eoin's situation. As we rose to leave, she looked at me gravely and said, "I'm concerned," then repeated, "I'm concerned."

On the way home, I focused my frustrations about Eoin's problems on this psychologist who could not provide an easy answer. What did her parting remark mean? Worry even if you do not know what you are worrying about? Have a good, unfocused anxiety attack?

I searched the local libraries for references to specific learning disabilities. The case histories I read bore minimal resemblance to Eoin, no more than they would have to a normal child.

Eoin's next appointment, nearly 2 months later, was in early December. After testing, the staff gave us a Christmas present of further uncertainty. No one could pinpoint Eoin's problem, but he did seem to exhibit "autistic-like behavior." We were told that someone on the staff would make an appointment for us at a diagnostic and treatment center at a university in a nearby town.

By mid-January, we had heard nothing about an appointment, so I telephoned the center and discovered that our referral had not been received. The woman I spoke with was pleasant but distant; she said that this agency worked only with autism and certain communication handicaps. Perhaps our son would be better served somewhere else. However, she did make an appointment for a diagnostic evaluation in May, the next possible opening.

The 4-month wait seemed interminable. We were relieved when another prospective client contracted chicken pox and we could fill his appointment on March 7. At the conference after the testing, no one specifically mentioned the word autism until I asked directly whether it applied to Eoin. The director said yes.

That pronouncement helped me stop evading the truth. We discussed Eoin's autistic characteristics, cited as difficulty in social relating, disordered and delayed language, inconsistent responses because of inability to process directions, and uneven development of skills. In imitation tasks, Eoin failed items at the 18-month level, but he succeeded in puzzles and matching and arranging tasks at the 4- to 5-year level.

The staff recommended that we begin using teaching activities daily with Eoin at home and return to the center weekly for the next few weeks. After that, we were to return for sessions every few weeks. Enrollment in preschool classes and private speech lessons came later.

OTHER REACTIONS

My husband and I did not broadcast Eoin's new label because we did not want people to shove him into a confining pigeonhole. We were also defensive, unsure how people would react. We did not want to admit that our child was not normal. It was hard enough thinking about autism and its ramifications for the future; discussing it would have made a nebulous concept painfully concrete.

Most of the handful of people we told were solicitous and consoling. A few others released barbs that stung for years. Had we been lax as parents? Had we played so much music that Eoin felt little desire to communicate in words? Had we disrupted his inner stability by moving several times in his early years? Had he lacked playmates? Had living in a bilingual area (Irish Gaelic and English) and speaking to him in both languages upset his linguistic equilibrium? Had John's frenetic schedule of work and school been a factor? At least no one called me a refrigerator mother.

FAMILY FEELINGS

Eoin was the first grandchild born to both sets of grandparents, so they were understandably thrilled at his arrival. Since the closest friends of John's parents had also been blessed with their first grandchild 6 months earlier, comparisons came naturally. I soon dreaded hearing about their child. She seemed like an obnoxious, supernatural prodigy as her accomplishments far outstripped Eoin's.

Just after Eoin's diagnosis, John's mother wrote us a loving, meticulously detailed analysis of Eoin's situation. She commented on 25 criteria presented in Lorna Wing's classic, *Autistic Children.* Only four of these characterized Eoin, she thought.

Gradually she began to accept his autism; she has since been very solicitous and supportive. Even so, we find ourselves ironically assuming a cautious parental role toward her when she reads about a promising new treatment or becomes overly optimistic about Eoin's progress.

Another relative provided a classic example of disappointment and denial of Eoin's autism. He said Eoin's problem was a lack of parental stimulation and discipline; he thought we allowed Eoin to do whatever he wanted. This relative suggested that we deny Eoin things if he did not say what was expected, and teach him words by constantly repeating them. My response finally was to send him one of the few angry letters I have ever written, in which I flatly said that he was wrong and I did not wish to discuss it further. At this point John and I realized that it was necessary to protect ourselves with a firm armor against criticism of our child or our childrearing methods.

SEARCH FOR SCHOOLING

I wanted to enter Eoin in the excellent seminary preschool, but was unsure how candid to be. I gave the director an honest appraisal of Eoin, backed by an encouraging letter from his therapist. The uncertainty and apprehension of wondering whether Eoin could attend the preschool was much greater than the anticipation of awaiting my own college acceptance. The director proposed a 2-week trial period, which became 2 happy, productive years spent in the 3- and 4-year-old classes.

Although his teachers had never before taught an autistic child, they willingly studied the two pages of notes I wrote on autism. We agreed that since Eoin's development was erratic, he would be placed a year behind his chronological age.

The teacher of the 4-year-old class was particularly sensitive to Eoin's needs because her own son had learning disabilities. When we asked her to write a letter to be used for kindergarten placement, she wrote:

> Eoin is loved and supported by all the other children, and he returns this love. He is not disruptive and understands and follows commands readily. When presented with a new activity, Eoin may appear not to want to do it. This is easily overcome by taking the activity to him— after you have let him watch you or the other children, e.g., put the brush in his hand and tell him to paint a picture. If you have Eoin's trust you have his cooperation.
>
> Eoin is a very special person... He has blended in well with our class and has been a definite asset.

We had the opposite experience when we looked for a kindergarten. We had moved 20 miles for John to assume a pastorate. Since we decided that large public school kindergarten classes would be untenable, friends recommended a private kindergarten near our house.

After I discussed Eoin's autism with the director, she grudgingly agreed to accept him for a 2-week trial. She did not assign him to the popular, patient, experienced teacher our friends had been pleased with, but to one who was young, inexperienced, uninterested in challenges, and who treated Eoin coldly and distantly, almost fearfully.

After a few days, she informed me that Eoin could not talk at all, but merely made noises; that he could not form his letters or draw a recognizable figure, but simply scribbled. I was surprised and disappointed because Eoin performed these tasks fairly well at home.

We endured the full 2 weeks because Eoin seemed contented. He like the playground equipment and enjoyed having the other children around him. I persuaded myself that if we persevered, Eoin might be assigned to the sympathetic teacher. Instead, we were told that Eoin was too handicapped to enter that school.

After an exhaustive search of all of the options in our area, we enrolled Eoin in private kindergarten 23 miles away. It was the best we could find for him, but it was not good enough. The teachers at the school were loving and accepting but their educational philosophy did not include the structure and encouragement an autistic child needs. By spring, they agreed with me that Eoin was happy but learning very little there.

As Eoin reached elementary school age, his deficits became more obvious. We discovered the Catch-22 of autism: Eoin is too handicapped to be normal, but too normal to be handicapped.

High-level autistic children are hard to place. The autistic classrooms in our county school system were geared to low-functioning children and were not appropriate. Normal classrooms were too large, and keeping up would have been impossible for Eoin.

For a time Eoin was placed in what was termed a "non-categorical self-contained" classroom. I privately referred to it as "the leftovers": a hodgepodge of too many children with too many differing handicaps and little common ground for learning together. Eoin was the only autistic child in the class.

Legislation about appropriate education seemed like a mockery to us; the school system's version of what was appropriate was a far cry from ours.

Placing Eoin in school continued to be a headache. By his third year past preschool, Eoin attended his third school. Despite the disappointments of the previous 2 years, we finally felt hopeful. His new class was the first in the county for high-functioning autistic children. For the first time, we could tell that he was actually learning something at school.

SOCIAL RELATIONS

One neighbor avoided us after I told her Eoin was autistic. "The autistic leper," I bitterly reflected, and decided to be even more discreet. We found it was not necessary in everyday life to reveal Eoin's autism. People in the supermarket or library simply saw an attractive, normal-looking child. True, he did not return their greetings, but many children are shy. He occasionally shouted inappropriately, but young children are forgiven such outbursts.

We knew we were fortunate that our child's behavior was not wild or disruptive in public. I admit that I often played a mental game when out with Eoin: Could he pass as normal? I watched other people react to him. Did they notice anything unusual? If not, ten points, Did they appear to think he was a normal child who just needed discipline? Six or seven points. Did they think he was weird? Zero.

Eoin's normally placid behavior in public has changed in recent months. He is becoming more extroverted, yet does not know how to articulate his wants or frustrations; shouting, shoving, or breaking something may be the result. In addition, periods of overflow energy may well up into an inappropriate outburst.

The uncertainty of knowing how Eoin will respond to a social situation is stressful, but I find my embarrassment quota rising as I become less sensitive to observers' opinions.

Supportive, understanding friends have been very helpful in dealing with Eoin's social inadequacies. I am grateful that our best friends are not put off by Eoin's peculiarities, but appreciate his sweet smile, his offbeat sense of humor, and his tentative expressions of affection.

A person's acceptance and affection for Eoin have inadvertently become criteria for friendship. I find myself immediately drawn to people who are interested in him. I do not expect them to be experts on autism, but I do appreciate it when they greet our son in a friendly way and tactfully ask how they can help him relate to them.

SIBLING RELATIONSHIPS

My husband and I decided to discuss Eoin's autism with people who needed to know because they dealt with him regularly. However, we never talked about autism in front of Lia or Conor, born when Eoin was 4. We wanted them to think of Eoin as their brother, not their brother the autistic person.

Some people dread telling their children about the "birds and the bees." Telling Lia and Conor about Eoin's autism seemed much more difficult to me. We decided to wait for questions and then provide short but honest answers.

Eoin's siblings grew up used to daily home programs and their brother's weekly trips to the speech therapist. They were accustomed to a brother who smiled but generally seemed to ignore them, who was normally sweet and gentle, but was rigid and obsessive as well. That was their norm. The long-awaited question did not arise until Lia was nearly 6. She informed me that she saw no point in asking Eoin questions because a neighbor's child had told her that he was retarded. I briefly said that was not true and explained his handicap, but we did not dwell on it.

Eoin's sister and brother have accepted his peculiarities because they have grown up with them. The three have worked out their own territories and modes of operation. The younger two are close companions; it does not usually occur to them to include Eoin in their play. We are pleased to see that they are becoming more thoughtful in that respect, and are even more pleased when he accepts their invitations rather than becoming withdrawn or anxious.

Conor, our youngest, is very gregarious. Eoin cannot retreat when Conor decides to tickle or tackle him, or insists that Eoin participate in some activity Conor has devised. Sometimes these demands irritate or anger Eoin. Since he does not yet articulate his frustrations well, he occasionally pushes or hits the other children. It is hard to know how to prevent this and when to intervene.

Balancing the care of siblings with the needs of an autistic child is difficult. I spend an hour or an hour and a half afternoons working solely with Eoin, so his siblings naturally expect special attention as well. Since they can be quite vocal about their demands, it is easy to neglect Eoin's needs for theirs. It is hard not to seem to be playing favorites. Finding games and activities that all three can participate in alleviates some of the pressure.

Despite such difficulties, our response was highly affirmative to the parents of an autistic child who debated whether to risk having another child. Lia and Conor are Eoin's best therapists. Although he causes them some embarrassment and pain, he can also be fun for them to be with. We hope that their compassion for and understanding of people who are different are a natural outgrowth of their relationship with Eoin. And despite our love for Eoin, we find it rewarding to have normal children as well—children who are articulate, affectionate, and observant, and who follow those tiresome charts in the baby books.

SUPPORT SYSTEMS

Monthly sessions at the therapy center give us ideas for home therapy and for working out everyday problems that arise. The therapists' assessments and suggestions motivate and encourage me; it is easy to become discouraged without having outside advice to draw on.

Five years ago the center first sponsored a trial eight-session mothers' group that has since become an institution. Behavior management is the perennially favorite topic, followed by social behavior and teaching techniques. A wide range of topics is covered, such as community resources, summer camp, sibling relationships, social skills programs, and current theories on autism.

Outside speakers who address the group provide valuable information, but when it comes to the nuts and bolts of daily life, the insights of the other mothers are invaluable. By pooling our collective experience, we usually arrive at workable suggestions for each other's problems.

As parents, we have a tremendous advantage over the experts. We know autistic children intimately. We know what they are like beyond the two-way mirrors. We eat with them, bathe them, play with them, are irritated and amused by them. We know that some theories do not hold water in real life. We also know that the best therapists cannot really know what our lives are like. We are buoyed by the confidence of knowing that we are progressing, if not triumphing.

The mothers in our group share a rare bond. Our meeting room is one place where we do not need to explain about or apologize for our

children. We can commiserate about the follies of school systems or let
down our guard enough to see the lighter side of our children's fixa-
tions on toilets or stop signs.

Until recently, parents of autistic children walked a lonely road.
This has changed greatly even since our son was diagnosed. In our
area, we can attend a countywide support group organized by parents
and participate in a county program that provides frequent workshops
and sets up parent-to-parent contacts. The state autism society is a good
avenue for lobbying for better programs for people with autism. Some
families also find the Association for Retarded Citizens helpful.

I have become selective in order to avoid becoming a victim of
support groups. Supporting support groups can subtract valuable time
needed for the autistic child or the rest of the family or even the parents
themselves. I have been chastised by other parents for not being more
active in the evening support group that meets once a month. Its programs are geared primarily to fairly handicapped children; their needs
and goals are not the same as ours. I sympathize, but rarely attend.

Our church has been a primary support for our family. The loving
acceptance and solicitous attention we have found there form a wel-
come oasis from a less caring world.

PARENTAL ROLES

Parents of autistic children assume roles not normally needed in
parenthood. At Eoin's birth we did not realize we would eventually
become researchers, therapists, and advocates.

Reading was my immediate reaction to Eoin's diagnosis. I vora-
ciously ploughed through every article and book I found about autism.
At my request, our therapist provided copious articles, which I sat up
late at night to read.

At first I was too uninformed and anxious to separate the mediocre
articles from the good, except to realize that some were terribly technical and boring. I was inordinately sensitive to what I was reading,
accepting all negative theories as fact and feeling wildly hopeful about
proposed cures: megavitamins, purines, allergies, etc. Hope springs
eternal with each passing fad. Eventually I attained an equilibrium that
permitted me to read and react more rationally.

As his therapist, I have the advantage of being the person Eoin knows and works with best. Working with him has forced me to improve my teaching skills. I am constantly challenged to find new approaches and break tasks down into simple, logical steps. How does one learn to button a button? It took days to master, with the aid of a huge, homemade buttonhole and the biggest button on hand. How do people tie their shoes? I wrote out directions for Eoin to read and follow.

How can we communicate with a person who "tunes out" much of what he hears? We learned to pare down our language and use familiar catchphrases when necessary.

In Lewis Carroll's *Through the Looking Glass,* young Alice finds herself being pulled along at breakneck speed by the Red Queen. Alice is nearly exhausted from frantic running when the queen finally allows her to rest.

> Alice looked round her in great surprise. "Why, I do believe we've been under this tree all the time! Everything's just as it was!"
>
> "Of course it is," said the Queen: "What would you have it?"
>
> "Well, in our country," said Alice, still panting a little, "you'd generally get to somewhere else—if you ran very fast for a long time, as we've been doing."
>
> "A slow sort of country!" said the Queen. "Now, here, you see, it takes all the running you can do, to keep in the same place. If you want to get somewhere else, you must run at least twice as fast as that." (p. 151)

So it is with the autistic child. When I feel as if we are catching up to Eoin's peers in one area, I discover that they have surged ahead in another. No matter how fast we run, we sometimes seem to find ourselves back under Alice's tree. I remind myself that we are not all running in the same race, but making comparisons comes easily and naturally.

ADVOCACY

Although current legislation and new programs have brought vast improvements in possibilities for young children with autism, parents still need to work hard to find the best situations for their children. We found that we could not sit on our hands and wait for good things to happen.

As advocates, we observed direct applications of tired truisms:

The buck does stop here, with us. The squeaky wheel does indeed get the grease when you are trying to get the ear of a school administrator or legislator. Go to the top if you want to get somewhere. Take things as they come.

Parents' input can be very influential in determining class makeup for the next year. Assertiveness has never been my strong point, but buttonholing members of the school system's department for exceptional children now comes naturally.

Keeping up with the bureaucracies is a part of parental advocacy. Eoin's many records and test scores seem to be all-important to administrators, yet this information was lost regularly in Eoin's transfers to new schools. I have been teased for lugging a huge tote bag to conferences, but no one laughed when I was the only person able to locate the necessary reports.

ADJUSTMENTS

Adjusting to having a handicapped child is a grieving process, for parents are grieving the loss of normalcy. For some time I attempted to deny my doubts about Eoin's difficulties and shortcomings. Even after he had been diagnosed and we had the reports on paper, it was hard to accept that strangers could have made an accurate, if devastating, assessment of him. For some time I had to force myself to read Eoin's diagnostic reports.

I felt some guilt about my childrearing, but not about childbearing. I had been so cautious during pregnancy that even our parents had kidded me a bit. No caffeine, no alcohol, no medication, no preservatives—nothing that seemed potentially harmful had passed my lips. Now it was ironically evident that all the extra grams of protein I ingested to give our child a good brain had not prevented this particular malfunctioning within his head.

Having an autistic child has not shaken my faith. I believe that God gives us the strength to help Eoin. I realize there are many worse tragedies than having an autistic child. My initial anger that Eoin had this problem shifted to occasional bouts of self-pity and daydreams that he would suddenly become normal.

A mother of another autistic child recently asked whether I fully accept our child's autism. I started to reply that I did, but then thought again. Sometimes I cannot bear to watch the rocking and antisocial behavior of a friend's Down syndrome autistic daughter because I do not want to see links between her handicap and Eoin's. Another friend helps with an autistic adult social skills group. I am not ready for that; the social awkwardness and disabilities of these young people would depress me. My honest reply had to be maybe.

It is hard to assess my own feelings. I remember coming to the parents' open house at Eoin's new school last fall. Although the school board had written us a letter assigning Eoin there, no one seemed aware of it. The office staff and teachers had never heard of Eoin, and of course had none of his records. All of my past uncertainty about where Eoin should be and how he would fare suddenly overwhelmed me and I felt helpless. I stopped in the hallway for a few minutes, as if waiting for someone to rescue me. But I am the one called on to do the rescuing, to figure out and straighten out and plod onward.

My grasp on what I consider an appropriate attitude is tenuous. At times I am discouraged and think, "Why bother?" I feel as if Eoin is drifting so far from us and everyone else that we may as well relax and let him be contented in his happy, self-made world.

At other times I feel nearly manic, aggressively attacking, intervening, encouraging, demonstrating. During these periods, visits to the autism center serve as a "fix." On the way home from these sessions, I chastise myself for all my shortcomings and vow to do better.

DAILY TENSIONS

Trying to fit a square peg into a round hole is a constant strain. How much should we push Eoin to meet the standards most of us live by? When do we intervene and when do we leave him alone?

Many deficit areas improve as an autistic child grows older, but lack of social skills becomes increasingly obvious. Refusing to speak, throwing tantrums, and shouting are considered normal for a 3-year-old; these behaviors stand out as abnormal a few years later. Should we force our child to take part in games at a birthday party? Must he respond to the mail carrier's pleasantries? When must we explain his behavior to strangers who are confused or critical? Sometimes my judgment defines the standards for behavior; at other times they are dictated by my fatigue.

Eoin's perseverative behavior taxes the whole family even when others are not present. His echolalic speech can be a wearing, slow torture. To varying degrees, everyone in the family is aware of Eoin's little and big compulsions and rituals and the reactions that will occur if they are not honored.

Uncertainty about Eoin's abilities, needs, and potential is an endless stress. What should we be doing for him? What should we be planning for the future? What kind of person will he be? What sort of life can we expect for him?

My attitudes fluctuate with my son's. His periods of poorer functioning are hard on me and the entire family. His good times are mine as well. I elevate my spirits with success stories of autistic people who have sufficiently overcome their handicap to live independent, productive lives. Even if this does not happen to our son, I live with the hope that it might.

Last fall a contingent from our mothers' group sat together at the state autism society's annual conference. We listened attentively as one speaker concluded with a parent's perspective: "Celebrate with me. Rejoice in who he is and who he will become, but forgive me if, from time to time, I shed a tear for who he might have been" (Bristol, 1987).

I watched the other mothers. As if by group reflex, every one of them dabbed at eyes that had been dry seconds before. Then I realized that my own eyes were too full to see very clearly.

ADVICE TO OTHER PARENTS

When I reflect on our son's early years, I find that I was guilty of playing the ostrich. I offer this advice to parents who suspect that their child is autistic: Do not bury your head in the sand. Do not imagine the problem will disappear if you ignore it. If your child consistently exhibits behavior that you consider abnormal, take him to good diagnosticians. Do not be placated by well-meaning friends or family doctors not trained to make such judgments. If you disagree with the first opinion, get a second or a third.

If the diagnosis is autism, do your homework. Read all you can find in local and university libraries. Send for materials and book lists from local and state autism societies. Become your child's best teacher. Find a regular place and time to work with your child in daily structured activities. Find out what services your school system offers that are geared specifically for children with autism, not for children with other disabilities.

In some parts of the world you may encounter ignorance or even hostility. Educate the educators. Help teachers understand how best to work with your child. Be imaginative and constructive in presenting alternative ideas to your child's teacher or the school system's special education division. Sometimes your ideas will be appreciated and used.

Find out about suitable physical, occupational, and speech therapy. If the school cannot provide therapy, find an agency that can. Check to see whether your health insurance will help cover costs and find clinics that charge according to income levels.

Ask the local "Y," or recreation department, or health club to offer a special swimming or gymnastics class for a small group of autistic children. Find out about local day camps and summer camps for children with autism.

Remember that others are in the same situation. Join a support group and become close to a few people in it.

Find a church or synagogue that offers loving acceptance as well as spiritual sustenance. Do not be discouraged if you do not find it at the first place you visit; just keep looking.

At times the demands of an autistic child can seem overwhelming. Take a break—spend an evening out, call a friend, read a book.

Be patient with yourself and with your child. Remember that all children are trying at times. Remind yourself of your child's good qualities and talents. Appreciate the child for what he or she really is rather than dwelling on what the child is not.

REFERENCES

Carroll, L. (1974). *Through the looking glass and what Alice found there*. London: Bodley Head.
Bristol, M. M. (1987, November). *What you should know about my child*. Paper presented at the Annual Meeting of the Autism Society of North Carolina, Durham, NC.
Wing, L. (1980). *Autistic children: A guide for parents*. London: Constable.

3

Normal Childhood Development from Birth to Five Years

ROGER D. COX

INTRODUCTION

The first 5 years of life are a time of remarkable change in the competence and independence of children. From a state of almost total helplessness, neonates quickly develop capacities needed to function more independently. Babies soon learn to organize information about their world and to signal and respond to signals. With time, they learn to move through their world without help, exploring it and then retreating to the security of laps or knees of parents or other caregivers.

By the time preschool-aged children are ready to start kindergarten, an amazing period of physical, cognitive, and social-emotional development has taken place. Average 4- to 5-year-old children run, jump, climb, hop, skip, gallop and occasionally crash on their way through the world. They can talk, sing, charm, tease, lecture, negotiate, resist, plead, and promise—depending, of course, on their mood at the moment. In addition to all of these skills, children use a complex language system involving lengthy verbal utterances created spontaneously and almost effortlessly. By age 5, children have learned to feel secure, to be afraid, to know anger and resentment, and hopefully, to

ROGER D. COX • Division TEACCH, Department of Psychiatry, University of North Carolina at Chapel Hill, Chapel Hill, North Carolina 27599-7180.

Preschool Issues in Autism, edited by Eric Schopler *et al.* Plenum Press, New York, 1993.

experience reciprocal love with parents and significant others of all ages. They have learned to hoard, share, resist and assist, and to laugh and cry alone and with others. Although more years of parental support will follow, a child about to begin kindergarten is ready for the challenges and excitement of consistent educational and social experiences beyond the family unit. Each fall parents of beginning kindergarten children shake their heads in amazement as their children are launched on a voyage of life experience, marked in many societies by the start of formal education.

This chapter presents some of the more important aspects of development during the typical child's first 5 years of development. Because it is not possible to describe or discuss in detail all developmental milestones, the focus is on the developmental accomplishments that allow children to function socially and to communicate within their world.

The newborn baby comes into the world needing care and attention to meet almost all of its life-sustaining needs. Infants are unable to reach or point with any precision, nor can they move around their environment by crawling for months after birth. Yet in a few short months, it becomes possible to observe surprising competencies in the young infant. These competencies are particularly impressive when we realize that, compared to time spent sleeping or nearly sleeping, the infant spends relatively little time in a state of arousal conducive to social interactions and new learning.

Watching a newborn infant for any length of time soon makes any observer aware of the baby's cycles of alertness, activity, quietness, and sleep. Even early in development, babies seem to be responding to more than just the signals of their environment. They seem to be responding to internal forces that regulate behavior and control in the receptivity to stimuli (Schaffer, 1977). Infant states that have been described include regular sleep, irregular sleep (sleep with writhing, stirring, and facial expressions), drowsiness, alert inactivity (alert and visually interested but quiet), waking activity (diffuse motor activity involving the whole body), and crying (Wolff, 1966). It is interesting to note that only alert inactivity is ideal for infant learning and infant-adult social interactions. But the newborn is capable of making use of even limited opportunities for learning and soon the infant is able to spend more and longer periods of time awake, alert, and ready to learn about the world. As that occurs, the child begins to achieve important developmental milestones.

MOTOR DEVELOPMENT

Infancy through Toddlerhood

Perhaps the most obvious change that one can see during the early development of the child is in the area of motor skills (Bayley, 1968; Malina, 1986). In a short span of time, an infant develops from a relatively helpless creature in need of constant care and attention to a toddler capable of walking alone. During the first 18 months of life, a child goes through an impressive progression of developing motor skills. Motor development occurs in a systematic and regular way, allowing the baby increasing capacity for more precise forms of movement.

The direction of motor development is described as moving from the head to the toes and from the center of the body to the extremities. Thus, the baby is able to lift its head up early, followed by raising its chest, with lower extremity control following these early milestones. At the same time, it is interesting to note how early in development interest in the hands occurs, with playing with the toes following later.

Although an early type of reaching and grasping is seen in the first month of a baby's life, controlled reach and grasp behaviors are not usually well-established until the sixth or seventh month. Early reaching does not accurately separate reaching and grasping, and although some success may occur, the coordination of reach followed by grasp is not well established. Also, this early reaching does not seem to be a well-coordinated effort between the eyes and the hand. That is, in the first month, early reaching efforts are not correctable by the child if the reach goes off in the wrong direction.

The development of reaching and grasping becomes well-developed by the sixth or seventh month as both motor control, tactile response, and visual systems are all able to work together. So the child is now able to see an object, reach for it with some precision and self-correction, and grasp it securely after touching it.

Three through Five Years Old

By age 3, there is a marked change in the child's independence and competence in motor activities. The 3-year-old child runs with a more fluid gait than before, starts and stops quickly, and can speed up and slow down with greater control. Stairs are climbed more easily, and the child is able to alternate feet while climbing. Jumping is better controlled because the child has the ability to jump with both feet together providing a better base for landing. Earlier jumps involved a leading foot so that landing was on one foot. The 3-year-old is able to stand on one foot briefly. It is time for the three-wheeler, and a little Big Wheel for many 3-year-old children now replaces the push and coast scooter used in the past.

During the next 2 years comes even better physical performance. Climbing, swinging independently, and better balance are all seen in the next 2 to 3 years. Skipping and hopping become a part of outside activities, and with the rise in these skills comes increasing self-confidence about activities that involve movement. Although the full complement of skills needed for coordinated ball-throwing or basketball bouncing have not yet developed, most of the running, jumping, and balancing skills used in simple forms of athletic activities such as track and field and artistic expression such as dancing are present by age 5.

Motor Development and Autism

Although children with autism have a number of pervasive development problems, the development of motor abilities in autistic children is usually within the normal range. In fact, since the motor development of a young autistic child is often a peak skills area, it is difficult for parents to monitor their child's behavior. Autistic children are often able to walk and move independently in their world without developing a sense of danger or cautiousness that helps protect the average child.

COGNITIVE DEVELOPMENT

Infancy through Toddlerhood

Cognitive development is one of the most important areas of development in the infant and toddler's life (Flavell, 1977). In fact, many of the important accomplishments in the areas of social and communicative development rely heavily on the child's mastery of certain cognitive skills.

During the first 2 years of a child's life, cognitive abilities are focused on the child's understanding of the relationship between external stimuli and/or internal states and motor movements. In the first year of life, the young child spends a lot of time learning to make responses that have effects. The baby learns to nurse more efficiently from the bottle or from the mother's breast. The baby learns to hold a rattle, then to shake it to make a noise. Complexity increases as the baby learns how to look for a toy that falls off the table or a ball that rolls away. Piaget (1954, 1967) described these motor developments as examples of sensorimotor learning (Piaget's first state of cognitive development).

Other developments that involve the relationship between motor behavior and objects include important skills for the child. Banging objects together is often an early sign of cause and effect understanding. Soon, the child is able to use objects and containers to "put in" and "take out." Later in the first year, the child begins to understand how objects fit into slots or form boards. This fascination with perceptual-organizational tasks can be appreciated best by scanning the shelves at toy stores for materials recommended for the child beginning at 6 to 9 months through more advanced perceptual-organizational tasks up through age 2 years.

During year two, the next broad period of cognitive development is marked by the use of language and symbolic function. One of the most important cognitive skills acquired during the preoperational stage of development (Piaget, 1954, 1967) is object constancy. Young babies seem unable to understand that the same object can appear in different places. They also seem unable to understand that objects covered from view can appear in the same place when uncovered. The relationship between where objects appear and the required movement to get them there is also a mystery to the young child. But starting at the end of the sensorimotor period (around 18 months) and throughout the preoperational stage of cognitive development, children learn the relationships between the permanence of objects, the spatial location of objects, and the movement necessary to change the locations of objects (Sugarman, 1982, 1983).

Three through Five Years Old

What began as an emerging ability to use language and symbolic thought during the latter part of the second year of life develops into a more sophisticated understanding of the world during years 3 to 5 (Fenson, Vella, & Kennedy, 1989). During the sensorimotor stage of development, the child's motor responses and actual manipulations of objects were the primary ways of understanding the world. From ages 3 to 5, children begin to understand their world in more symbolic ways expressed through language and a beginning understanding of abstract concepts. Thinking seems to be primarily static during the preschool years, focusing on a single feature at a time. Therefore, it is often difficult for children to hold multiple dimensions of objects in mind while solving problems. It is possible, though, for the preschool child to understand that some things "go together" so that a primitive type of conceptual sorting is possible. Because thinking during this period is egocentric, it is often difficult for the child to explain things clearly to others. In spite of the limits of this type of thought, the ability to begin to see groupings based on shared abstract qualities marks a major milestone in the child's development.

Cognitive Abilities in the Autistic Child

The relationship of autism to the development of cognitive, non-language skills is complex. It is generally recognized that a relatively high percentage of autistic children function in the range of intellectual abilities described by the term mental retardation. So, in the general sense, one would expect overall cognitive skills to be lower for an autistic child than for a normal child. However, with autistic children, the area of perceptual-organizational abilities, including the visual-motor skills needed to do puzzles and form boards, is often less impaired than other abilities. It is when cognitive development becomes more symbolic and less concrete, as in the development of language, that autistic children usually show major deficits.

SOCIAL AND EMOTIONAL DEVELOPMENT

Visual and Auditory Stimuli during Infancy and Toddlerhood

Even within the first 6 months of life, infants appear to be particularly interested in visually presented stimuli. And yet young infants do not attend equally to everything in their visual fields. Very young infants seem to prefer to look at representations of the human face. In fact, in one study, Fantz (1961) found that infants as young as 2 months of age spent more time visually fixated on a target resembling a human face than on any other patterned stimuli. This classic research has been extended in studies that show a developmental shift in the scanning of real faces (Haith, Bergman, & Moore, 1977). Infants 3 to 5 weeks old fixated on the presented face only 22% of the time. Infants of 7, and 9 to 11 months old fixated on the face 88% and 90% of the time, respectively. Moreover, the older infants spent less time looking at the contours of the face and more time looking at the eyes. These researchers concluded that the eyes probably become meaningful to infants as a focus of social interaction some time between age 5 and 7 weeks, and that infants' increasing eye contact and focus on faces in general are important in the development of the social bond between child and caretaker.

It is more than just the visual representation of the human face that attracts and pleases the infant. Not only do infants like to look at the human face, but as soon as they can give a real smile, the face and voice are the best stimuli one can present to elicit a smile. Before 3 weeks of age, only incomplete or partial smiles can be elicited from infants, but at about 3 weeks, full-blown smiles involving the infant's whole face start to occur. The auditory stimulus most effective in eliciting these smiles is the sound of the human voice (particularly the female voice), and the most effective visual stimulus is a representation of the human face (Kaye & Vogel, 1980).

It may not be the human per se that infants respond to in smiling (Sroufe & Waters, 1977). In fact, it has been shown that a crude mask with lines for a nose and mouth and blackened circles for eyes will work to make babies smile. T. G. R. Bower (1979) reported that even a plain piece of cardboard with two eyelike blobs will elicit smiling. Some theorists use such findings to suggest that it is certainly not a recognition of shared humanness that causes infants to smile at cardboard with "eyes," but it seems important to acknowledge the strong predisposition that infants seem to have to recognize and respond to eye-like stimuli. In fact, it even has been demonstrated that a card with numerous pairs of dots will elicit more smiling than will a card with a single pair of dots. So, one can argue that it is the contrasts that the infant is smiling at, not a real face. Even though technically this may be correct, what is clear is that infants come into the world particularly attuned to the sights and sounds associated with their human caregivers.

Early Social Interactions: Imitation Skills in Infants

Even if one tried to discount the interest that infants have in human faces and voices, there is also evidence that even very young infants are capable of and interested in simple imitative actions with caregivers. It was also assumed until fairly recently that the actions needed to imitate developed relatively late in infancy and that a highly sophisticated cognitive structure was necessary for imitation to occur. However, the capacity for imitation appears to be available within the first few weeks of life (Melzoff & Moore, 1977). Infants in Melzoff and Moore's study were observed to imitate adults in opening the mouth, puckering the lips, widening the eyes, opening the hand, moving the fingers, and sticking out the tongue. The mutuality of these imitative actions does seem to indicate that specific body parts of the adult are recognized in some primitive way by the infant. The interactive nature of this imitative game can also be reversed with adults imitating infants, with the infants showing rapt attention when the adult does so, and the imitated actions increasing in frequency. Therefore, it seems that this imitative game with young infants does indeed qualify as an early stage of social behavior, though it probably does not satisfy a definition of communicative behavior (Bower, 1979).

Imitation is one indication that infants are capable of social interaction at an early age. However, even hours after birth, interactional or communicational synchrony has been observed in newborns. This term refers to the motor behavior shown by the infant when spoken to by an adult. Both speaker and listener move together in a very subtle dance-like manner, with the rhythm of the dance coming from the cadence of the spoken words. What this communicates, of course, can be the source of some discussion, for it does not seem that there is a message communicated by the infant. As Bower (1979) states,

> interactional synchrony transmits no precise messages but rather a degree of togetherness, rapport, participation, nonisolation, which is exactly the base required for an I-thou relation. The behavior is specifically human; in infants it can be elicited by human speech and no other auditory stimulus. (p. 306)

Toddlers and Their Attachment to Primary Caregivers

When infants begin to be able to move about their environment through crawling and creeping, early signs of social interest and social responsiveness are reflected in the universally observed phenomena of separation anxiety and attachment behavior. The terms *attachment* and *attachment theory* have come to have special meaning due, in large part, to the pioneering work of Bowlby (1958, 1969).

Three distinct developmental abilities are necessary in order for attachment to occur. First, object constancy must have occurred within the cognitive process. As described earlier, object constancy refers to the child's ability to realize that when a perceived object is no longer present in the immediate vicinity, it still exists. Obviously the memory must be sufficiently developed to allow for a mental representation of objects and people. But more than just memory is required. The infant must know that something present and then absent still exists and can be sought out and potentially rediscovered. Second, it seems to be no coincidence that the occurrence of attachment corresponds to the rapidly developing ability of the young child to move about through one or more forms of self-propulsion. As infants learn to control muscles to allow rolling, then creeping and crawling, and finally erect walking, the development of attachment also is occurring. Third, attachment is more than just an evolutionary protective mechanism. It is an expression of the strong sense of sociability of the developing child. Bowlby (1958, 1969) has argued that the normal processes of perceptual development help the child understand that the mother figure is distinct and different from strangers. Bowlby (1969) also has described in detail how the child develops a fear of new or strange things, including strange people. Thus, fear or anxiety response plays a major role in the development of attachment. Attachment to people and places combined with fear of the unknown work within a group of behavioral systems that maintain a steady state between an individual and the environment (Bowlby, 1969; Bretherton, 1985).

In simple terms then, attachment and fear of the unknown combine to provide a counterforce to the system which encourages exploration or other forms of stimulus seeking behavior. When interest in exploration takes the child away from a primary attachment figure, stress, anxiety, and fear move the child back toward an attachment figure. When the world is safe and reasonably well known, the child's developing physical ability and interest in the environment lead to exploring and moving away. When stressful situations arise (as when strangers enter the room), attachment pulls the child back physically closer to attachment figures.

Attachment research has been conducted to provide an empirical study of the importance of the bond that develops between mothers and their toddlers (Lamb, Thompson, Gardner, & Charnov, 1985; Radke-Yarrow, Cummings, Kuczynski, & Chapman, 1985). The most frequently used experimental paradigm in attachment research is the "Strange Situation," a standard series of eight episodes involving separations and reunions between mothers (and more recently, fathers) and their young children. Although the initial interest in developing the "Strange Situation" was the exploration behavior of the young child when the mother was absent from the room (Ainsworth & Wittig, 1969), the differing response patterns of the children during reunion episodes with the mother turned out to be of particular interest. Many children responded as expected with distress at the mother's leaving and active seeking of physical contact at her return. Some children who had not become distressed at the mother's leaving still greeted her and actively sought interaction and engagement with her when she returned. Other children showed a very different pattern when the mother returned. One interesting group of children showed angry, resistant behavior mixed with positive attachment behavior, giving observers the impression of children with highly ambivalent feelings toward their mothers. Another group of children appeared to avoid or ignore the mother upon her return. As a group, these children not only were not distressed by separation from their mother, but they did not actively seek out reunions with her. Recently, another type of child, characterized by disorganization and disorientation upon reunion, has been described (Main & Solomon, 1986).

The interpretation of those various attachment patterns in nonhandicapped children has undergone considerable change in recent years. Initially, because attachment theory was historically based on the effects of maternal deprivation in children, explanations for why there are different attachment patterns focused on the characteristics of the mother. As expected, it is possible to identify maternal characteristics that account for some of the differences in both optimal and nonoptimal attachments (Radke-Yarrow *et al.,* 1985). More recent research, however, has begun to examine the important characteristics that the infant brings to the mother-child relationship in the development of attachment with the mother. While the active investigation of parental and infant characteristics that contribute to secure attachment continues, it seems that researchers have developed increasingly complex models of the interactive relationships between good parenting and infant capabilities that result in secure and insecure attachments (Sroufe, 1985).

Beyond Attachment: Play in the Preschool Child

Play has its origins in the first year of life. Early sensorimotor play, primarily undertaken for the pleasure that the activity brings, soon is replaced by shared activities that involve playmates. As children grow and develop, the relationship with primary caregivers is supplanted by the peer relationships that develop around the activity of play. Through the development of successful play skills, children experience the beginnings of friendship patterns (Giffin, 1984; Gottman, 1983; Lewis, 1982; Lewis, Feiring, & Brooks-Gunn, 1987).

Infants begin to respond to their peers early in the first year of life (Vandell, Wilson, & Buchanan, 1980). When placed close to each other, gazing can be seen for an extended period of time even with 2 or 3 babies 2 to 3 months old. Touching soon follows, and by the end of the middle of the first year, approaches, following, or other gestures designed to increase interactions have been observed. Certainly, anyone who has visited a McDonald's playground is aware of the high interest, imitation, and early game playing such as run and chase that develop by 12 to 18 months of age. With familiar peers, even sharing toys is observed shortly after 12 months. Such positive exchanges increase during the second year as well, though aggressive and antisocial behaviors are also seen to increase (Cummings, Iannotti, & Zahn-Waxler, 1989).

When children enter the preoperational stage of development (approximately age 2 years), play begins to be more symbolic. Because they can use symbolic thought, children soon use language in developing fantasy situations in their play. Imaginary playmates are but one example of this in children's play. Additionally, play during the preoperational phase of development allows children to engage safely in role playing. Children can become doctors, lawyers, dancers, cowhands, or any desired character simply by donning the appropriate costume and announcing their intentions. Role-playing allows children to practice being authority figures like parents or teachers in safe, nonthreatening situations.

The progression of infant-to-infant play behaviors has been described as falling into a three-stage developmental sequence (Mueller & Lucus, 1975; Mueller & Vandell, 1979). During the first stage, described as objected-centered, infants tend to cluster around a toy with most of their attention on the toy and with little or no attention given to each other. During the second, or simple interactive stage, the children respond to the behavior or peers. This stage is marked by one child attempting to regulate the behavior of another, almost as if the second child were an object. An example from the work of Mueller and Lucus (1975) nicely describes this type of interaction.

> Larry sits on the floor and Bernie turns and looks toward him. Bernie waves his hand and says "da," still looking at Larry. He repeats the vocalization three times more before Larry laughs. Bernie vocalizes again and Larry laughs again. The same sequence of one child saying "da" and the other laughing is repeated 12 more times before Bernie walks off. (p. 224)

In the third stage, the complementary interactive stage, the behavior of the infants becomes more complex and sequences of social interchanges occur. Imitation becomes more common and reciprocal and complementary role reversals begin. Children take turns being the one chasing and the one chased. They alternate being the giver and the receiver. It is this stage of development, the complementary interactive stage, marked by flexibility of roles and reciprocity, that provides the basis for later close interpersonal relationships. By this third stage, children's interactions are marked by the sense of mutuality. Along with ability and interest in this type of interaction with peers comes a decrease in the intensity of the attachment relationship.

How can we explain the decrease of interest in parental interactions which occurs with the increase in peer relationships even in preschoolers? Bower (1979) suggested that the shift from attachment to peer relationships is much easier to understand if we think of the child as having a basic drive to communicate with others. The growing sense of communication skills and the ability to have mutuality occurs most readily when there is a match between the child and others who can share the same world view. The shift in interest is somewhat natural when one understands that as children grow and begin to use language, adults begin to reject or attempt to modify statements that indicate childish thoughts. Peers who have a similar worldview accept the statements of the young child without adultlike criticism, making it understandable for the child to learn to prefer peer interactions (Bower, 1979).

Social and Emotional Development and Autism

Children with autism have problems with social and emotional development. All aspects of development described in this section are likely to show problems. Autistic children typically do not show an understanding of early imitation, nor are they likely to have appropriate attachment relationships with primary caregivers. Their play is marked by repetitive, stereotyped behavior patterns that are often nonfunctional and difficult to interrupt. Though it is sometimes possible to teach autistic preschoolers to engage in a form of parallel play, the extent to which they remain aloof from others around them is significant. Though some high-functioning autistic preschool-age children may show some imaginative play, it is usually limited in its occurrence and is highly repetitive in nature.

LANGUAGE AND COMMUNICATION

Infancy through Toddlerhood

One of the most outstanding achievements of the child is the mastering of language. Even before language develops, average children already have begun to communicate wants and needs to significant others. Body positioning, eye contact accompanied by facial expressions, gestures, and even temper tantrums all can be considered forms of communication that do not involve language. With normally developing children these early forms of communication are supplemented quickly by spoken language. Though not the primary form of communication for very long, these early communicative responses are important because they form the foundation for later symbolic communication through language.

Although language has a complex system of rules, all normally developing children learn to understand and use language in a very short period of time. Because children do seem to have a special interest in communicating with others from early in their development, language quickly becomes a preferred method of both giving and receiving information. The functions of language are numerous, and children quickly learn to use all aspects of language. Halliday (1975) suggested the following 7 functions for language.

1. Instrumental. Language enables us to satisfy needs and express wishes. This is the "I want" function.
2. Regulatory. Through language we are able to control the behavior of others. This is the "do that" function.
3. Interpersonal. Language can be used for interacting with others. This is the "me and you" function.
4. Personal. We express our own unique views, feelings, and attitudes through language. We establish our personal identity through language.
5. Heuristic. After we begin to distinguish ourselves from our environment as children, we use language to explore and understand the environment. This is the question-asking function, the "tell me why" function.
6. Imaginative. Language permits us to escape from reality into a

universe of our own making. This is the "let's pretend" or poetic function of language.

7. Informative. We can communicate new information through language. This is the "I've got something to tell you" function.

Children are remarkably adept at using both expressive and receptive language from early in their development. Although the spoken word is not usually present until the end of the child's first year, a clear pattern of development leads up to it. Beginning at birth, children cry. Vocalizations such as cooing follow, often starting in the first month of the baby's life. Babbling, beginning in the middle of the first year, quickly comes to have a strong resemblance to adult speech in inflection, rhythm, and tone. Finally, patterned speech, typically in the form of single-word utterances, occurs at the end of the first year (Kaplan & Kaplan, 1970).

Early speech is in the form of one-word utterances. The most common form used is the label, which children use to name objects. Other categories of words are action words (e.g., *give, bye-bye*), modifying words (e.g., *red, dirty*), personal and social words (e.g., *yes, no, please*), and function words (e.g., *more*). Children do not use words with the full adult sense of the word meaning, however. Initially words are used in a highly restrictive way with a word only used to name a particular object. Later, a child may overgeneralize, using a word like doggie to refer to all four-legged animals. Early language development seems to be a time for hypothesis testing for the child, with the adult listener used to help refine the use of the words.

Using two-word utterances usually occurs at about 18 to 20 months, although there is considerable variability in this. Children in many countries learning their own native language use two-word utterances in a highly similar way. Utterances showing relationships such as recurrence (e.g., *more milk*), attributive (*big ball*), possessive (*mama sock*), action-locative (*walk street*), agent-action (*doggie go*), action-object (*hit ball*), and question (*where ball*) have been reported universally in children's early two-word use of language. To understand the specific use of language, it is necessary at this stage of development to have the context in which the child uses the words. Children often use the same two-word utterance to mean more than one thing at this time. For example, "mommy sock" may mean "Mommy, give me the sock" or "that's Mommy's sock," depending on the context.

Children soon begin to use strings of words and break out of the pattern of two-word utterances. From the ages of 2 to 3 years, language typically undergoes a remarkable transformation. The length and complexity of children's utterances increase, and children begin to use more complex sentences to convey information to others. Children's imitations remain linked to their developmental level, so that a sentence with too much complexity will be repeated at a child's own current level of ability. That is, the sentence, "Give me the red ball" may be repeated as "give ball," "give me ball," or "give me red ball," depending on the child's level of development. When the child omits words, they are those containing the least information. So the completeness of the repetition is not random, nor based on the child's ability to remember the most recent words best (i.e., short-term memory), but seems to reflect an analysis of meaning even in early, less complete repetitions (Gleitman & Wanner, 1982).

Three through Five Years Old

Mistakes continue as children 4 and even 5 years of age try to understand both the rules of language and the exceptions to the rules. However, while the subtleties of language are far from learned, the ability to use words to communicate almost all types of messages to adults and other children is present. The development of plurals, tenses in verbs, and the use of interrogative words have all been studied in terms of young children's language errors. But by age 4 to 5, the ability to give and receive information is impressive. Examine this brief story that a 4-year-old recently told me and that I typed out verbatim. It illustrates some errors the child makes and shows how the themes of fantasy, relatedness, helpfulness, and emotional reactions are all included by a child in this age range.

> There once was a bad pony, and he wished he had a girlfriend. But he did not have a girlfriend, and he would always go off in the meadow or the forest or the field and look and look. But he would never find a girlfriend. And one day, out in the field, when he went out, there was standing another pony and she was crying and crying. Then this little pony, who was a girl, tried to fly but her wing was broken. And she told him to take her back to the castle so she could get it fixed. And then she hopped onto his back and he rode her off. When they got back to the house, the king was real mad. Because when he saw the princess he sent

the prince to the dungeon and he sent her out. Then she got him out and she rode from the king's guards who lay by the dungeon who were fast asleep. The end.

Language and Communication Development and Autism

Autistic preschool-aged children are typically unable to use language and communication skills appropriately. Language is often very slow to develop, and when it does, it is usually atypical in form. Repetitive, sing-song qualities of voice are often observed, along with the tendency to repeat phrases heard previously without evidence of comprehension. This repeating, called echolalia, is sometimes immediate and sometimes delayed. Both language and communication are affected by autism, and even the high-functioning autistic child usually displays oddities in language development and use.

SUMMARY AND DISCUSSION

The study of normal development from infancy through the preschool years has had a major impact on the understanding of autism. Autism is now considered a pervasive developmental disorder in diagnostic nomenclature (American Psychiatric Association, 1987). The term *pervasive* accurately reflects the fact that autism has an effect across all areas of psychologic functioning. To study and understand the disorder of autism, researchers and clinicians alike have started with the knowledge base acquired through the study of normal development. This chapter has focused on some, but certainly not all, of the important and relevant milestones of normal development.

The study of autism is at the earliest stages of development, spurred on by the emergence of developmental psychopathology (Cicchetti, 1989). This volume will attempt to provide new information on the interface between normal development and autism with a focus on the first 4 to 5 years of life. In the past, many important contributions in understanding autism have been made by researchers who came to the field of developmental psychopathology with backgrounds in all areas of normal developmental psychology, including social-emotional development, linguistics and psycholinguistics, cognitive development, and perceptual development. Because autism affects the interrelationships between development in all these areas, the challenge of understanding autism remains formidable. It is encouraging, however, to see from the contributions to this volume the promise of future developments in understanding autism.

REFERENCES

Ainsworth, M. D. S., & Wittig, B. (1969). Attachment and exploratory behavior of one-year-olds in a strange situation. In B. M. Foss (Ed.), *Determinants of infant behavior* (Vol. 4, pp. 111–136). New York: Wiley.

American Psychiatric Association. (1987). *Diagnostic and statistical manual of mental disorders* (3rd ed., rev.). Washington, DC: Author.

Bayley, N. (1968). *Bayley's scales of infant development.* New York: Psychological Corporation.

Bower, T. G. R. (1979). *Human development.* San Francisco: Freeman.

Bowlby, J. (1958). The nature of the child's tie to his mother. *International Journal of Psycho-analysis, 39,* 350–373.

Bowlby, J. (1969). *Attachment and loss: Vol. 1. Attachment.* New York: Basic Books.

Bretherton, I. (1985). Attachment theory: Retrospect and prospect. In I. Bretherton & E. Waters (Eds.), *Growing points of attachment theory and research: Monographs of the Society for Research in Child Development, 50,* 3–18 (Whole number 201).

Cicchetti, D. (1989). Developmental psychopathology: Past, present, and future. In D. Cicchetti (Ed.), *The emergence of a discipline: Rochester symposium on developmental psychopathology* (pp. 1–13). Hillsdale, NJ: Erlbaum.

Cummings, E. M., Iannotti, R. J., & Zahn-Waxler, C. (1989). Aggression between peers in early childhood: Individual continuity and developmental change. *Child Development, 60,* 887–895.

Fantz, R. L. (1961). The origin of form perception. *Scientific American, 204,* 66–72.

Fenson, L., Vella, D., & Kennedy, M. (1989). Children's knowledge of thematic and taxonomic relations at two years of age. *Child Development, 60,* 911–919.

Flavell, J. H. (1977). *Cognitive Development.* Englewood Cliffs, NJ: Prentice-Hall.

Giffin, H. (1984). The coordination of meaning in the creation of a shared make-believe reality. In I. Bretherton (Ed.) *Symbolic play: The development of social understanding* (pp. 73–100). New York: Academic Press.

Gleitman, L., & Wanner, E. (1982). Language acquisition: The state of the state of the art. In E. Wanner & L. Gleitman (Eds.), *Language acquisition: State of the art* (pp. 3–48). New York: Cambridge University Press.

Gottman, J. M. (1983). How children become friends. *Monographs of the society for research in child development, 48* (Whole number 201).

Haith, M. M., Bergman, T., & Moore, M. J. (1977). Eye contact and face scanning in early infancy. *Science, 198,* 853–855.

Halliday, M. A. K. (1975). *Learning how to mean: Explorations in the development of language.* London: Arnold.

Kaye, K., & Vogel, A. (1980). The temporal structure of face-to-face communication between mothers and infants. *Developmental Psychology, 16,* 454–464.

Kaplan, E. L., & Kaplan, G. A. (1970). The prelinguistic child. In J. Eliot (Ed.), *Human development and cognitive processes.* New York: Holt, Rinehart & Winston.

Lamb, M. E., Thompson, R. H., Gardner, W., & Charnov, E. L. (1985). *Infant mother attachment:*

The origins and developmental significance of individual differences in strange situation behavior. Hillsdale, NJ: Erlbaum.

Lewis, M. (1982). The social network system: Toward a general theory of social development. In T. Fields (Ed.), *Review of human development* (Vol. 1, pp. 89–122). New York: Wiley.

Lewis, M., Feiring, C., & Brooks-Gunn, J. (1987). The social networks of children with and without handicaps: A developmental perspective. In S. Landesman & P. M. Vietze (Eds.) *Learning environments and mental retardation* (pp. 371–400). Washington DC: American Association on Mental Deficiency.

Main, M., & Solomon, J. (1986). Discovery of an insecure–disorganized/disoriented attachment pattern. In T. B. Brazelton & M. Yogman (Eds.), *Affective development in infancy* (pp. 95–124). Norwood, NJ: Ablex.

Malina, R. M. (1986). Physical growth and maturation. In V. Seefeldt (Ed.), *Physical activity and well-being.* Reston, VA: American Alliance for Health, Education, Recreation, and Dance.

Melzoff, A. N., & Moore, M. K. (1977). Imitation of facial and manual gestures. *Science, 198,* 75–80.

Mueller, E., & Lucas, J. (1975). A developmental analysis of peer interaction among toddlers. In M. Lewis & L. Rosenblum (Eds.), *Friendship and peer relations* (pp. 223–258). New York: Wiley.

Mueller, E., & Vandell, D. (1979). Infant–infant interaction. In J. D. Osofsky (Ed.), *Handbook of infant development* (pp. 591–622). New York: Wiley.

Piaget, J. (1954). *The origins of intelligence.* New York: Basic Books.

Piaget, J. (1967). *On the development of memory and identity: Heinz Werner lectures, Clark University, Worchester, Vol. 2.* Barre, MA: Barre.

Radke-Yarrow, M., Cummings, E. M., Kuczynski, L., & Chapman, M. (1985). Patterns of attachment in two- and three-year-olds in normal families and families with parental depression. *Child Development, 56,* 884–893.

Schaffer, R. (1977). *Mothering.* Cambridge, MA: Harvard University Press.

Sroufe, L. A. (1985). Attachment classification from the perspective of infant–caregiver relationship and infant temperament. *Child Development, 56,* 1–14.

Sroufe, L. A., & Waters, E. (1977). Attachment as an organizational construct. *Child Development, 47,* 1184–1199.

Sugarman, S. (1982). Developmental change in early representational intelligence: Evidence from spatial classification strategies and related verbal expressions. *Cognitive Psychology, 14,* 410–449.

Sugarman, S. (1983). *Children's early thought: Developments in Classification.* Cambridge, MA: Cambridge University Press.

Vandell, D., Wilson, K., & Buchanan, N. (1980). Peer interaction in the first year of life: An examination of its structure, content, and sensitivity to toys. *Child Development, 51,* 481–488.

Wolff, P. (1966). The causes, controls, and organization of behavior in the neonate. *Psychological Issues, 5,* 7–11.

II

Specific Aspects of Autism

4

Early Social Development in Autism

CATHERINE LORD

Social deficits may be the most long-lasting and handicapping aspects of autism (Park, 1986; Rumsey, Rapoport, & Sceery, 1985), but they are also the least well-documented in research. More encouraging, however, is that research on social deficits has increased significantly in the last 5 years, and, as it accumulates, we have had access to many vivid and remarkably similar clinical examples of the social difficulties of autistic people (Kanner, 1943; Wing, 1976). DSM-III-R, the diagnostic system in greatest current use in North America (American Psychiatric Association, 1987), in fact, consists of these examples supporting a very broad statement about a qualitative social deficit. However, to date, no comprehensive theory has been proposed that attempts to account for these examples over the course of development, although more specific accounts have been put forward (Frith, 1989; Hobson, in press).

Social behaviors can be described on many levels, and are affected by many nonsocial factors (Lord, 1990). Thus, it can be difficult to know where to begin to conceptualize the social problems of the young autistic child. Perhaps that is why, even though many professionals and parents of older children feel that social deficits are primary to the syndrome (Volkmar, 1987), social difficulties are not necessarily the first source of concern for parents of very young autis-

CATHERINE LORD • Department of Psychiatry, University of Chicago, Chicago, Illinois 60637.

Preschool Issues in Autism, edited by Eric Schopler *et al.* Plenum Press, New York, 1993.

tic children (Gillberg *et al.*, 1990; Le Couteur *et al.*, 1989). Volkmar (1987) pointed out that the social behavior of young autistic children is remarkable because of the contrast between it and the demanding, omnipresent sociability of most nonautistic toddlers and preschool children, and the contrast between the relative lack of concern shown by many autistic children over social encounters and the intense interest exhibited by the same children over trivial aspects of the physical environment. If the contrasting situations are unavailable, the lack of social behaviors of young autistic children may be more a source of confusion to a parent or nonexpert professional than clear diagnostic indicators.

Cohen, Paul, and Volkmar (1987) recently categorized the social deficits of autistic children as falling into three areas: sociability, attachments, and understanding and expressing emotions. In this review, I will use these categories plus one additional domain drawn from researchers of normal development (Hetherington, 1983)—behaviors related to social success (such as play and adaptive skills)—to describe the social behaviors of autistic children during preschool years. Though antisocial and aggressive behavior are considered to be part of social development, they will not be discussed here, since these difficulties are considered along with behavior problems in another chapter (Van Bourgondien, this volume). This review will describe methods of assessment of social behavior, and will conclude with a discussion of current interventions. Obviously, significant overlap exists between social and cognitive and social and communication deficits. Where issues are covered in detail elsewhere in this volume, they will be mentioned only briefly here (see Prizant & Wetherby, this volume).

SOCIABILITY

Sociability refers to a person's interest and ease in being with other people. For our purposes, we can further subdivide it into three subcategories: motivation and approaches, imitation, and social knowledge. Communication also belongs within this category, as well as several others, but is addressed in its own chapter (see Prizant & Wetherby, this volume).

Social Motivation and Approaches

While diagnostic criteria have included descriptions of a "pervasive lack of social awareness" in autistic children (American Psychiatric Association, 1980), a simple-minded conceptualization of the autistic child as having no social attention, interest, or motivation has generally not been supported by research or clinical reports. Numerous studies have shown that very young and school age autistic children generally look at people as frequently as do mental age-matched nonautistic peers and as frequently as they look at objects, at least in laboratory settings (Dawson, Hill, Spencer, Galpert, & Watson, 1990; Sigman & Mundy, 1989; Wetherby & Prutting, 1984). While the absolute number of directed gazes has been similar, in some cases the duration of gaze of autistic children was noted to be shorter both for looking at people and objects (Hermelin & O'Connor, 1970).

Three factors, however, seem to discriminate autistic children's attention to other people. First are attempts to avoid direct eye gaze or auditory input; such behaviors are extremely rare in normally developing or developmentally delayed children. (Kubicek, 1980; Wenar, Ruttenberg, Kalish-Weiss, & Wolf, 1986). Second is the infrequency with which autistic children try to attract other people's attention (Dawson & Galpert, 1986). Third are specific deficits in joint attention (Kasari, Sigman, Mundy, & Yirmiya, 1990; Loveland & Landry, 1986). Autistic children are less likely to follow another person's gaze or point to "share" attention to an object with someone else. Moreover, just because a child is looking at another person or even looking at whatever the other person is looking at does not mean that he or she shares an interest or even an awareness of the other person as a person or as having another perspective (Baron-Cohen, 1989). Diagnostic differences lie not so much in general attention to others or in simple social motivation, but in specific aspects of attention and in the behaviors from which it is inferred, such as changes in gaze and facial expression.

Imitation

Young autistic children's difficulties with motor and vocal imitation are well documented. Preschool and school-age autistic children have been found to show spontaneous motor imitation of others with less frequency and across a more limited range of behaviors than mental-aged matched peers (DeMyer *et al.,* 1972; Dawson & Adams, 1984) and to also be less adept at elicited imitation of gestures or familiar actions with objects (Bartak, Rutter, & Cox, 1975; Curcio, 1978). In fact, a recent study revealed that elicited imitation was the best discriminator between mental age-matched autistic and mentally handicapped preschool children out of a variety of measures of play and social skills (Stone, Lemanek, Fishel, Fernandez, & Altemeier, 1990). Imitation ability in autistic children has been found to be correlated with other social skills and with language level (Dawson & Adams, 1984; DeMyer *et al.,* 1972), but not with other early sensorimotor abilities such as object permanence (Curcio, 1978).

Social Knowledge

Relatively little is known about the social knowledge of autistic preschool children. We do know that, even as adolescents, autistic children have difficulty recognizing the sex and age of other people (Hobson, 1986; Weeks & Hobson, 1987). In contrast, a number of studies have shown no specific deficits in autistic children's recognition of their own reflections (Dawson & McKissick, 1984; Ferrari & Matthews, 1983; Spiker & Ricks, 1983). However, the ways in which autistic children behave when presented with their own reflections are often quite different from those of other children (Neuman & Hill, 1978); they do not show embarrassment or coyness. In an unpublished study that tested whether autistic children used a "probable event" strategy to help understand simple sentences, we found that school age autistic children had far less knowledge about social probable events, such as that mothers are more likely to wash babies than babies to wash mothers, than did normally developing 2-year-olds (Lord, 1985). It is easy to underestimate how much social knowledge most children have in the preschool years, but autistic preschoolers seem very likely to be significantly handicapped in this area.

ATTACHMENT AND RELATIONSHIPS

Relationships with Parents

Laboratory studies of attachment using the Ainsworth paradigm have shown that autistic preschool children have some attachment to their parents—they respond when left by a parent with a stranger, direct more behavior to a parent than to a stranger, and show changes in behavior upon reunion with a parent (Shapiro, Sherman, Calamari, & Koch, 1987; Sigman & Mundy, 1989; Sigman & Ungerer, 1984). However, as with motivation and attention, a closer look reveals differences in the quality of the autistic children's behavior. Autistic children are much less likely to respond to reunion by sharing or showing their parent something (Sigman & Mundy, 1989). The differences in quality and quantity between how the autistic children interact with their parents and with strangers are also smaller than for mentally handicapped or normally developing children of equivalent cognitive levels (Sigman & Mundy, 1989).

In contrast, most parents of autistic children retrospectively report concerns about their children's attachments to them (Le Couteur et al., 1989; Ohta, Nagai, Hara, & Sasaki, 1987). Diagnostic differences exist between autistic and mentally handicapped children as to whether or not their parents report their ever having experienced stranger or separation anxiety (Le Couteur et al., 1989), or accept affection from them (Van Berckelaer-Onnes, 1983). However, the degree of difference depends on whether parents are asked to describe behaviors that are associated with inferences of attachment and their feelings about these situations (in which case, most parents of autistic children indicate concern), or whether they are asked pointblank whether or not their child is attached to them (in which case most parents indicate their children are attached). This contradiction is an example of the importance in considering methods of assessment in interpreting conclusions about social behavior.

Most research with parents has used mothers only (Le Couteur et al., 1989), though in some cases mothers, fathers, and daytime caregivers have been treated as interchangeable (Sigman & Mundy, 1989). Differences between parents in how they behave with their autistic child and how the child behaves with them seem likely, given that a number of studies have shown that mothers often provide the bulk of direct care and also tend to feel more stressed by their children's difficulties (Konstantareas & Homatidis, 1989). In this same vein, it is interesting to note that parents of younger autistic children report less stress than parents of autistic adolescents and adults. Even more interesting is that the source of this stress is generally not social deficits, but rather, visible, embarrassing, or dangerous behaviors such as self-injury, inappropriate vocalizations, or stereotyped behaviors (Konstantareas & Homatidis, 1989).

Relationships with Siblings

Very little is known about autistic children's interactions with their siblings. Studies of siblings have tended to focus on the adjustment and cognitive skills of the other children in the family rather than how the children interact (Dunn, 1988; McHale & Gamble, 1986). One study looking at the spontaneous communication of school age autistic children showed great variability in the amount of time autistic children spent interacting with their siblings (O'Neill & Lord, 1982). This is an area that is difficult to study, but in which more information is greatly needed.

Relationships with Teachers

Clinical experience suggests that many young autistic children become very attached to their teachers; that is, they show distress if they are absent and signs of positive affect when they are together. One study with slightly older autistic children showed that the children communicated more when their teachers were actively working with them than in a less teacher-directed situation (McHale, Olley, & Marcus, 1981); however, structure, as well as the teachers' active engagement, was also a factor. One study of a preschool program for autistic children in which relationships between teachers and children were seen as a very important factor, showed the children made significant gains over those expected based on previous rates of progress, in social and language development (Rogers & Lewis, 1989). Given the number of autistic preschool children participating in educational programs, this seems like another area worthy of investigation.

UNDERSTANDING AND EXPRESSING EMOTION

Emotions can be expressed in many ways. By far, the greatest amount of research in the expression of emotion by autistic children concerned facial expressions. Most research about emotions has been carried out with older school-age or adolescent autistic subjects. Because of this distribution of information, I have devoted an entire section below to facial expressions of young autistic children and then grouped other modes of emotional expression and understanding and responding to others' emotions (across a variety of modes) together under one heading. The final section in this area concerns emotional arousal.

Facial Expressions in Young Autistic Children

Describing the facial expressions of autistic children has been an interesting, sequential process carried out over a number of studies in the last few years. Parents report that their children developed a social smile at a later age, show a more narrow range of facial expressions (Le Couteur et al., 1989), and show more frequent inappropriate facial expressions than do children of equivalent cognitive levels (Konstantareas & Homatidis, 1989). Yet the evidence from observational studies is more mixed. Kubicek (1980) and Massie and Rosenthal (1984) both found few facial expressions overall and particularly few positive expressions and smiles in studies of autistic children as infants and toddlers, interacting with their parents in relatively natural situations. Snow, Hertzig, and Shapiro (1987) found autistic preschool children to show fewer positive and more negative expressions than their classmates. These observations were carried out during relatively unstructured ordinary class time.

Even more interesting than the absolute amount of affect expressed was Snow and colleagues' finding that the autistic children's positive affect was far less likely than their classmates' to be socially directed. In two studies using semistructured interactions with an experimenter during a standardized social-communicative assessment (Mundy, Sigman, Ungerer, & Sherman, 1986), autistic preschool children were shown to have more "flat" or ambiguous facial expressions overall (Yirmiya, Kasari, Sigman, & Mundy, 1989), but to be particularly lacking in positive affect during episodes of joint attention (Kasari *et al.*, 1990). Another study observing autistic preschool children in semistructured interactions with their mothers showed no differences in the overall amount of smiling between the autistic children and mentally handicapped children, and few episodes of frowning in any of the children, but less reciprocal smiling between autistic children and their mothers and fewer smiles associated with eye contact (Dawson *et al.*, 1990). Thus, real differences in facial expressions do seem to be associated with autism, particularly in unstructured situations and in coordination with other socially-directed behaviors.

Expressing Emotions through Voice or Gesture

Parents of verbal autistic children of preschool age describe them as not showing normal vocal inflections associated with expression of feelings (Le Couteur *et al.*, 1989). However, this has not yet been documented in observational studies, in part because so many very young autistic children lack sufficient language skills for these judgments to be made. Older autistic children have also been described as using fewer emotional gestures (Attwood, Frith, & Hermelin, 1988) than mentally handicapped children. One of the difficulties in studying gestures, however, is that there tend to be large individual and contextual differences even within a normal population (Acredolo & Goodwyn, 1988; Attwood *et al.*, 1988; Lord & Magill, 1989) that make it very difficult to interpret the absence of gestures as abnormal without extensive normative data. Autistic children have also been described as expressing emotions, particularly excitement and frustration, in unusual ways, that often involve whole body or arm movements rather than the facial expressions or vocalizations seen in normally developing children (Carr, 1983).

Although clinical reports of unusual vocal expression abound, there has been relatively little systematic exploration of this area (Baltaxe & Guthrie, 1987). The one classic study is by Ricks (Ricks & Wing, 1976), in which parents of normally developing infants were able to identify the emotion expressed by all of the other normally developing children, but could not identify the voice of their own child;

whereas the parents of young, nonverbal autistic children could reliably pick out their own child and identify his or her emotion, but could not understand the emotions expressed by the other autistic children. This finding suggests that autistic children do have predictable ways of expressing emotions vocally, but they may be idiosyncratic and thus require learning to interpret as communication.

Understanding and Responding to the Emotions of Others

Most of the research concerning labeling and describing the emotions and internal states of others has been carried out with adolescents and young adults (Baron-Cohen, 1988; Hobson, in press; Hobson, Ouston & Lee, 1989). Even within this literature, results have suggested that the autism-specific deficit may not lie in giving verbal labels to emotional expressions (usually depicted in photographs, or by dolls, but sometimes conveyed through videotaped vignettes), but in comprehending more complex expressions of emotions and internal states that may involve the coordination of nonverbal and verbal behaviors (Hobson, 1990). With younger children, particularly nonverbal preschool age children, sufficiently sophisticated methods have not yet been employed to know much about what they do and do not understand, and the extent to which group differences are due to language or cognitive delays versus autism.

Parent report studies have indicated that parents of young autistic children describe them as less affectionate, less responsive to parental gestures of affection, and less likely to offer comfort than other children (Le Couteur et al., 1989; Ohta et al., 1987; Van Berckelaer-Onnes, 1983). However, as is true for attachment, how parents are asked about these behaviors makes a great difference (Stone & Lemanek, 1990). A number of studies have found frequent reports by parents that their children "use people as objects" (Dawson & Galpert, 1986; Knobloch & Pasamanick, 1975). Part of using people as objects has to do with children physically manipulating their parents' hands as they would tools, but an additional connotation is that children fail to show, while physically near or interacting with their parents, the emotional expressiveness that one would expect in a normally developing baby who is playing with his mother's hair or pulling at her skirt.

Emotional Arousal

A final aspect of emotion that has not yet been studied in detail, but for which interesting ideas have been raised, is emotional arousal. Recently, Dawson and Lewy (1989) suggested that many of the developmental difficulties of autistic children could be explained by a failure to take in certain kinds of information due to an overly high level of arousal that results in both excluding certain kinds of input and in attending to unusual stimuli. Clear evidence of this phenomenon in young children is not yet readily available, but case reports of frequent avoidance of eye contact in autistic infants (Kubicek, 1980; Massie & Rosenthal, 1984) could be used as support for it. In addition, parent's reports of irritable babies and difficulties in soothing young autistic children might also be related, though again the relationship between these behaviors and arousal might not necessarily be a simple one (Watson & Marcus, 1988).

BEHAVIORS AND SKILLS ASSOCIATED WITH SOCIAL INTERACTIONS

When parents and educators think about social skills, often what comes to mind are not just socially-directed behaviors, but also non-social behaviors that affect a child's social acceptability (Watson & Marcus, 1988). For the young autistic child, such skills fall in two general areas: play and adaptive skills.

Play

Numerous studies have shown that young autistic children show less appropriate functional play in unstructured situations (Mundy *et al.*, 1986; Sigman & Ungerer, 1984; Stone *et al.*, 1990) and less frequent and less complex symbolic play in structured situations (DeMyer, Mann, Tilton, & Loew, 1967; Mundy *et al.*, 1986; Sherman, Shapiro, & Glassman, 1983) than children of equivalent cognitive or language levels. One parent report study of autism in very young preschool children showed limited imaginative play to be one of the strongest indicators of autism (Dahlgren & Gillberg, 1989). Not only do many autistic children show limited imaginative play, but many also have intense and unusual interests in objects or sensations (Schopler, Reichler, & Renner, 1986).

The autistic child's difficulties in play are important, not just because of the insight they provide into his or her cognitive level, but also because they are associated with significant social limitations. Even those children who do engage in imaginative play at some level have great difficulty playing reciprocally with someone else (Harris, 1989; Leslie, 1987). This added difficulty has been interpreted primarily as the response to an increased cognitive demand. However, difficulties in play also have social consequences because they result in certain kinds of social opportunities not being available for autistic children, leaving the autistic child without the tools to participate in everyday social interactions with peers.

Adaptive Skills

Adaptive skills (such as toileting and feeding oneself and responding to "no") are part of social skills because their absence has real social implications and because they can have a significant effect upon a child's access to different social situations, from community playgroups to restaurants to visiting grandparents. A recent series of studies has provided very useful information about the adaptive skills of young adults with autism (Volkmar, Sparrow, Goudreau, Cicchetti, Paul, & Cohen, 1987), but relatively little is known about self-help and independence in autistic children. One recent study compared adaptive skills of autistic school-age children to those of older adolescents and to age-matched mentally handicapped children (Jacobson & Ackerman, 1990). During school age, overall scores for self-help skills of the autistic children were actually better than for the comparison group, but not during adolescence and adulthood. As adults, autistic people still surpassed mentally handicapped people in skills requiring gross motor abilities and in toileting, but they were not as competent as the mentally handicapped group in other areas.

Clinical experience suggests wide variability among young autistic children and within each child in self-help skills (Watson & Marcus, 1988). Many autistic children seem almost precocious in self-help activities that have a clear, meaningful result for them, such as opening containers, taking off their clothes, and operating video equipment. A substantial minority of autistic children almost toilet train themselves and are able to obtain food at relatively age-appropriate times. On the other hand, there are autistic children who are very difficult to toilet train, and others who require very systematic teaching in order to feed themselves.

One social issue that arises during the preschool years that affects self-help skills in normally developing children is the desire to be "grown-up." Normally developing 3- and 4-year-olds see their parents and siblings taking care of themselves and want to be like them. They may be embarrassed if they behave in a way that they feel is typical of a younger child. This motivation is not a factor for most autistic children until they are significantly older, but it leaves parents having to provide much more direct teaching about these behaviors, and in some cases, providing more direct consequences for these behaviors than would be necessary for other children.

ASSESSMENT OF SOCIAL BEHAVIORS IN AUTISM

Assessment of social behaviors in autism is usually done for two reasons: (1) to determine a diagnosis and (2) to measure an individual child's skills and behaviors in order to assess progress, set goals and design interventions or educational programs. In most cases, specific instruments do not accomplish these goals directly for social behavior in the way that a language test would yield particular scores and suggest specific aspects of communication that the child might be ready to learn. Together, the Autism Diagnostic Interview (Le Couteur *et al.*, 1989; Rutter, Le Couteur, Lord, 1990) and the Vineland Adaptive Behavior Scale (Sparrow, Balla, & Cicchetti, 1984) probably come closest to accomplishing these goals through parent report. The Autism Diagnostic Interview is a semistructured, investigator-based interview that focuses on parents' descriptions of children's behavior in social as well as other areas. It is designed for the purpose of making a diagnosis, but also provides a good sense of how a child behaves in ordinary circumstances and his or her parents' perceptions of his or her behaviors. The Vineland Adaptive Behavior Scale is a well-standardized parent interview that provides scores in socialization, communication, self-help skills and motor abilities. However, because of the variability in normally developing young children's behaviors, it often seems to yield very low age equivalents and rather high standardized scores for autistic preschoolers. Thus, the scores can be difficult to interpret, although the specific information about what the child does not do at home and in the community is often very useful.

The Autism Diagnostic Observation Schedule, a standardized schedule for the assessment of the social and communicative behavior of autistic children in which an examiner plays with and talks to the child following a semistructured protocol, has also recently been developed for children with verbal-mental ages of about 3 years and up (Lord, Rutter, Goode, Heemsbergen, Jordan, & Mawhood, 1989). This obviously excludes most autistic preschoolers. Work is in progress to develop a version appropriate for younger and/or nonverbal children. In the meantime, many of the general instruments, particularly the Psychoeducational Profile Revised version (Schopler, Reichler, Bashford, Lansing, & Marcus, 1990), offer good opportunities for observation of social behaviors. The Childhood Autism Rating Scale provides several useful social ratings as part of a more general diagnostic instrument (Schopler *et al.*, 1986).

Thus, in this section, rather than further describing assessment instruments that are well-covered elsewhere (see Marcus & Stone, this volume), two issues will be discussed in the assessment of social behavior in very young autistic children: how to determine what social deficits are specific to autism, and how to separate children's responses to structure and routine from spontaneous, social behaviors.

Identifying Primary Social Deficits versus Secondary Social Problems

Most young children referred for developmental evaluations are not autistic (Chess & Rosenberg, 1974). Referrals for "autistic behavior" include children with mental retardation and/or a variety of neurologic and sensory impairments (Gillberg *et al.*, 1990; Knobloch & Pasamanick, 1975), or communication deficits and odd behaviors associated with social anxiety or extreme activity levels (Dahl, Cohen, & Provence, 1986; Levine & Demb, 1987; Rescorla, 1988).

Even without autism, significant cognitive delays may affect a child's recognition of others' emotions and the child's flexibility in responding to these emotions (Brownell, 1986). For example, mentally

handicapped children are reportedly slower to smile (Cicchetti & Serafica, 1981) and have more difficulty labeling emotions than normally
developing children (Hobson, 1986). A child may also fail to show
particular normal social behaviors because of specific difficulties in
motor functioning, anxiety, or hyperactivity (Cohen, Paul, & Volkmar
1987), particularly when these difficulties occur in combination with
communication delays. For example, a very active child may not take
the time to seek comfort from his or her parent when hurt. A child with
significant motor delays may also fail to seek comfort because he or
she is not easily mobile (Watson & Marcus, 1988). In neither case is
the child necessarily autistic.

Because one goal of assessment is to identify autism-specific social deficits, it becomes important to first try to rule out other possible
explanations for concerns about a young child's social behavior (Rutter,
1985). In order to do this, clinicians need to be familiar with situations
and behaviors that are clearly associated with the consistent lack of
reciprocal social interaction that is part of autism, as opposed to those
that are affected by other sorts of problems. The quality of the behavior
must be considered, as well as its frequency or absence. If we are going
to depend on qualitative judgments of social behavior to discriminate
autism, we must be sure of both what the range of normal qualities of
behaviors in the relevant situations are, and the range of autism-specific
qualities. In many cases, this information is not available on standardized tests.

From this point of view, when working with young children, the
most important source of information is the parents. Questions may be
most useful when they address specific everyday situations that parents
can describe in sufficient detail so the clinician can make a judgment
about the quality of the child's behavior (Le Couteur et al., 1989).
Parents can be very accurate in describing real examples of behavior
(Schopler & Reichler, 1972), even though they may have difficulty
making overall judgments of whether or not their child is abnormal
(Le Couteur et al., 1989). It is interesting to note that, when a scale
designed to describe school-age autistic children was given to parents
of normally developing children, most normal children passed all the
social items by 3 months of age (Wenar et al., 1986). Thus, when
questions are asked in certain ways, the overlap between autistic children and a population of normally developing infants and preschool

children is minimal. On the other hand, when questions requiring yes or no responses are asked, and/or when the comparison group includes children with any other sort of disorder, the overlap becomes much greater (Dahlgren & Gillberg, 1989).

Masking of Social Deficits by Structure and Routine

A second concern in assessing social factors in autism is the potential failure of parents or professionals to recognize social problems because of the structure and initiative taken by parents in interacting with infants and very young children (Kasari, Sigman, Mundy, & Yirmiya, 1988). It can be difficult, particularly for parents, to recognize emotional detachment in a child when the mother and father automatically interact with him or her in an exaggerated, stimulating and structured way (Adrien, Ornitz, Barthelmy, Sauvage, & LeLord, 1987; Ohta et al., 1987; Volkmar, 1987). Parents may be more likely to perceive a child who treats people as objects as abnormal, than a child who usually ignores people completely, but who responds if tickled or tossed in the air.

Studies have suggested that shared attention between normally developing infants and their mothers is more often due to mothers following their children's gaze than vice versa (Collis & Schaffer, 1975). Likewise, because they offer comfort automatically, parents may not realize that a child does not spontaneously come to them, particularly if the child is never let out of their sight. This may be one reason why parents of younger autistic children tend to rate them as less severely abnormal, in comparison to professional ratings, than parents of older children, even though parents of younger children describe themselves as more stressed by specific behaviors (Bebko, Konstantareas, & Springer, 1987; Konstantareas & Homatidis, 1989).

Observations of the child, particularly with his or her mother, may be most useful in assessing autism-related social deficits, if they focus on the child's overtures and approaches, and if they can occur during unstructured times, as opposed to mother-dominated play or in response to formal contexts such as the strange situation paradigm. Observations of the child's behavior in more structured activities led by the mother can be very useful in providing an impression of how the parent is coping and in suggesting further interventions, but not so much in diagnosis.

As noted earlier, older preschool-aged autistic children have been shown to respond to separation from their mothers (Shapiro, *et al.*, 1987) and to seek proximity in this situation (Sigman & Ungerer, 1984; Sigman & Mundy, 1989). Therefore, the presence of some attachment-like behavior is not a contraindication to autism. The focus of observations and interviews might more appropriately be specific deficits in the child's attempts to elicit joint attention, in the child's emotional expressiveness during shared activities, in reciprocal social smiling, and in the number of approaches to mothers during unstructured play that have discriminated young autistic children from other groups of children (Baron-Cohen, 1989; Loveland & Landry, 1986; Snow *et al.*, 1987).

Given many parents' difficulties in recognizing early social deficits, parental concerns about a lack of attachment or being treated as an object must be taken very seriously (Ohta *et al.*, 1987). For parents who have not noticed a lack of reciprocity in their child, it can be difficult for them to know how their child would behave if they, the parents, were not as intrusive (Lord *et al.*, 1983; Lord & Magill, 1989). A child's negative or subdued reaction to unfamiliar, unstructured social situations created during an assessment may be attributed, in part correctly, to unfamiliarity, rather than to autism-specific deficits. A further difficulty is that the social behavior of very young nonautistic children may be even more disrupted than that of an autistic child in unfamiliar situations. Thus, identifying appropriate situations for observation and discussion during interviews will depend on accumulation of findings from well-designed research projects with appropriate control groups.

One option would be to observe the child with an adult who is familiar, but who is less likely than the mother to provide a highly structured environment in which to interact. The obvious candidate is the father, though grandparents, full-time babysitters, other relatives, or close family friends may also be appropriate. Research with normally developing infants (Lamb, 1977) and toddlers (Clarke-Stewart, 1978) has shown children under 3 years to often be more positive and more cooperative with their fathers than their mothers during play, even though these fathers and children spent considerably less time together than mothers and children. One might suspect that these differences would not be the same for many young autistic children, and that abnormalities in social behavior, such as minimal responsiveness, little or unusual eye contact, and rare attempts to share enjoyment or play might be more easily observed during young autistic children's interactions with their fathers (particularly if roughhousing and tickling are placed temporarily off-limits) than with their mothers. After a diagnostically oriented observation, however, it may be wise to let parents interact with their child in whatever way they like, including physical play, so that one has the opportunity to also observe the child at his or her best.

With older autistic children, the diagnostic importance of considering social behavior with peers has been suggested (Lord, 1984; Wing, 1976). In fact, if one had opportunities for lengthy observations and to provide all preschoolers with equivalent peer experiences, deficits in peer interaction should be even more obvious in autistic children when they are very young, than at school age. However, because of practicalities, this is generally not possible. Marked lack of interest in other children is one characteristic of autism that can be determined, even in toddlers and preschool children who have had relatively little experience with peers (Cohen *et al.*, 1987; Ornitz, Guthrie & Farley, 1977). Most nonautistic young children show a definite interest in other children, whether in a grocery store or a playground or on television, that does not seem to be based on experience. In preschool children who have had frequent opportunities to play with the *same* other children, a lack of pretend play *with* other children seems to be the deficit most specifically associated with autism, although the information currently available is limited, and the ability of this measure to differentiate autistic children from severely mentally handicapped children during the preschool years has not yet been supported (Leslie, 1987; Ungerer & Sigman, 1981). Hesitancy around groups of other children and difficult behavior (including mild aggression) toward peers, and quantitative measures of complementary-reciprocal play, such as chasing, are not particularly stable characteristics even in normally developing children (Howes, 1987). Thus, we would expect these factors to be less useful in discriminating autistic children than lack of interest and the inability to pretend in a social context.

Behavior with siblings, particularly a complete lack of interest in an older sibling, is also a potential source of information about social deviance (Lewis, 1987). However, because of differences in family size, birth order, intervals between births, and family interaction patterns, a child's lack of interest in a sibling, especially a very young preschool child's lack of affection or concern about an infant brother or sister, is not unusual (Parke & Tinsley, 1987).

Other possibly diagnostic social behaviors are probably best directly observed as the child interacts with a stranger who can deliberately manipulate the kinds and amount of social structure he or she is imposing (Lord *et al.*, 1989; Mundy *et al.*, 1986; Schopler *et al.*, 1990). Normally developing children often use more overt nonverbal behaviors with a stranger than with a caregiver (Podrouzek & Furrow, 1988). However, clinical observations suggest that even autistic children who show some response to a parent may be relatively indifferent to an unfamiliar adult who does not deliberately structure or intrude on their behavior (Watson & Marcus, 1988). In this case, the clinician has the opportunity to make specific adjustments in his or her behavior (Shapiro, Frosch, & Arnold, 1987) and to deliberately vary the structure of the interaction (Clark & Rutter, 1977; Schopler, 1976; Volkmar & Cohen, 1988). The effects of these adjustments on the child's responsiveness, ability to take turns, play cooperatively, and communicate expressively can be observed.

A summary of suggestions for assessment is provided in Table 4-1. In order to avoid confusing social deficits related to general mental handicap or other factors with those specific to autism and in order to avoid overestimating a child's sociability because of the structure provided by his or her parents in their everyday routines, it is critical to acquire information in a variety of ways about a child's behaviors across different contexts and with different people. As shown in Table 4-1, a child's interest and ability to spontaneously approach and seek interaction may be best judged by direct observation with his or her mother. Responsiveness and social flexibility may be better measured on the basis of detailed descriptions or observations of interactions with fathers or other familiar adults. Specific nonverbal and verbal behaviors (such as social referencing) may be best observed in semistructured interactions with a clinician.

TREATMENT OF SOCIAL DEFICITS

Treatment of social deficits will be considered in four sections. First, traditional approaches to treatment will be discussed briefly. Sec-

Table 4-1. Proposed Social Characteristics of Young Children with Autism

Behavior or Deficit Most Likely	Method of Determination
Rare or limited spontaneous social approaches when there is no need for help (Baron-Cohen, 1989; Mundy et al., 1986)	Observation with mother; parental report
Rare or limited seeking of or response to attempts to establish joint attention to objects (Loveland & Landry, 1986; Mundy et al., 1986)	Observation with mother; parental report
Rare or limited sharing of positive emotion regarding specific actions or events (Snow et al., 1987; Gillberg et al., 1990)	Observation with mother; structured observation with clinician; parental report
Limited flexibility in responding to nonphysical play behaviors and lack of attempt to sustain them (Shapiro et al., 1987; Stone & Lemanek, 1990)	Observation with father or familiar adult; parental report
Limited responsiveness, as indicated by vocal play and nonverbal communication, particularly eye contact and changes in facial expression, to adults other than mother (Kasari et al., 1988; Stone & Lemanak, 1990)	Observation with father or familiar adult; structured observation with clinician; parental report
Possible, but Less Likely or More Difficult to Observe	
Failure to offer comfort (Le Couteur et al., 1989)	Parental report
Lack of "automatic" interest in unfamiliar children (Cohen et al., 1987; Ornitz et al., 1977)	Parental report
Lack of reciprocal, pretend play with other children (Lord & Hopkins, 1986; Strain & Cooke, 1976)	Parental report
Lack of interest in an older sibling (O'Neill & Lord, 1982)	Parental report; observation with sibling
Parental concerns about lack of attachment or treating people as objects (Ohta et al., 1987)	Parental report; observation with mother

ond, how and where treatment occurs will be addressed. Third, questions about selecting behaviors to be targeted for intervention will be raised. Fourth, a summary of general issues in treatment will provide the conclusion.

Approaches to Treatment of Social Deficits

Three main approaches to treatment may be considered separately, though in fact almost all intervention programs use principles from each of them. The behavioral approach emphasizes teaching according to basic principles of learning including contingency and contiguity (Dyer & Peck, 1987). In recent years, behavioral approaches in education have changed substantially to involve more natural antecedents and consequences and more frequent incidental teaching. Programs tend to be less data-oriented, though theoretically data should still be used in all decision-making. The range of behaviors targeted and taught has expanded considerably (Donnellan & Kilman, 1986).

A developmental approach addresses treatment of social deficits from a somewhat different perspective, though often the methods used are directly derived from behaviorism. A developmental approach assumes that learning will be easier and more easily generalized if goals are determined by following a hierarchy of sequentially acquired skills seen in normal development. In addition, there is an assumption that behavior changes may follow a child's increased understanding of a concept or situation and do not have to be directly trained in all cases (Dawson & Galpert, 1986; Dyer & Peck, 1987).

The third approach, the ecological approach, also employs aspects of the other two perspectives, but emphasizes goals of participating in normal day-to-day community functions. The focus is on goals that are immediately useful for the child and on working on these goals using age-appropriate tasks in least-restrictive environments (Dyer & Peck, 1987). For young children, this includes a focus on integration into community preschool programs.

Where and How Treatment Occurs

Residential programs for preschool children are very rare now and are primarily aimed at obtaining thorough diagnoses of complex behavioral and medical problems. Still, sometimes parents of newly diagnosed children wonder if a 24-hour program would be better than typical day programs, and hence may pursue residential treatment. In fact, not only is there no evidence that residential programs are more effective than outpatient or home-based treatment, there is some evidence that they are less effective (Sherman, Barker, Lorimer, Swinson & Factor, 1988). Residential treatment is particularly poor at producing progress that can be generalized (Lovaas, Koegel, Simmons, & Long, 1973). Helping parents find alternative placements when they feel unable to cope or short-term respite care when they need a break, are important issues, given the scarcity of good foster homes and respite care, but need to be considered separately from residential treatment justified for the sake of the child.

Home-based treatment has been used with autistic children for over 20 years (Anderson, Avery, DiPietro, Edwards, & Christian, 1987; Howlin, Cantwell, Marchant, Berger, & Rutter, 1973; Howlin & Rutter, 1987). Home-based treatment has been shown to be effective in increasing children's social behaviors and in changing the ways in which parents interact with their children. In one study, these changes have been shown to be superior to those experienced by children who were participating in traditional preschool programs, although it is not clear exactly what these programs were (Anderson et al., 1987). Another recent study directly compared home-based to outpatient treatment of preschool and early school-age children and found little difference in the results, with both methods superior to residential treatment (Sherman et al., 1988). There seems to be relatively little disagreement about the benefits of seeing parents and children in their own homes; however, because of the cost of home-based programs and the lack of clear evidence of their superiority, there has been a general move back to clinic-based treatment, with regular home visits incorporated as part of the assessment and treatment plan (Schopler, 1989).

Outpatient treatment of young autistic children's social difficulties tends to be of two sorts: parent-oriented and preschool treatment programs. Often these approaches are offered as a joint service, or at least with coordinated consultation among different programs (Rogers & Lewis, 1989; Schopler, 1989). When parent training has been contrasted to direct outpatient treatment by individual therapists (not in a preschool), working with parents has been shown to be much more effective (Koegel, Schreibman, Britten, Burke, & O'Neill, 1982). Family work emphasizes parents as cotherapists (Schopler, 1989) and teaching parents principles of behavior management (Schreibman, 1988). Psychodynamic or family systems approaches have not been shown to be useful in improving the social behaviors of autistic children.

Preschool programs vary on a continuum of specialization from integrated community programs to cross-categorical programs to special classes for young autistic children (see Lord, Bristol, & Schopler, this volume). Direct comparisons of these programs are not available, but all have shown improvements in a variety of communicative, social, and self-help skills (Harris, Handleman, Kristoff, Bass, & Gordon, 1990; McEvoy, et al., 1988; Odom & Strain, 1986; Rogers, & Lewis, 1989). Three programs particularly well-known for their organization and innovative approaches are the Denver and New York Hospital programs, which emphasize a developmental approach to communication and affective development (Rogers & Lewis, 1989; Shapiro *et al.*, 1987; Snow *et al.*, 1987), the Rutgers Program, which is more behavioral (Harris *et al.*, 1990), and LEAP (Learning Experiences . . . An Alternative Program for Preschoolers and Parents; Hoyson, Jamison, & Strain, 1984), which contains an excellent peer-training module for integrated classrooms. The TEACCH preschool classroom model is also described in detail in this volume (Lord, Bristol, & Schopler, this volume).

Social Behaviors Targeted for Intervention

Behaviors targeted for intervention will be considered under the same headings in which the social deficits specific to autism were discussed at the beginning of this chapter: sociability, including imitation and social approaches; relationships and affect, which will be considered together; and skills that underlie social interactions, including play and adaptive behaviors.

Treatment of Deficits in Sociability

The two social behaviors most frequently targeted for change have been amount of interaction and imitation. Many behavioral studies have shown treatments yielding increased amounts of interaction, usually between autistic children and normally developing children, rather than family members or other handicapped children (McEvoy *et al.*, 1988; Odom & Strain, 1986). In general, these have not been particularly robust findings. That is, significant amounts of prompting of either the autistic or the nonhandicapped child are often necessary to maintain gains and it has not been clear how much the improvements have been due to changes in the normally developing playmates rather than the autistic children. Often, there has been relatively little generalization. In our work with school-age children, the behavioral procedures and training with playmates that resulted in the most marked changes in amount of interaction also resulted in substantially less generalization over time and across partners than did interventions in which the normally developing peers were allowed to behave more naturally (Lord, 1984;

Lord & Hopkins, 1986). However, situations may be different with younger children.

Overall, increasing the amount of time that young autistic children spend interacting through changing the behaviors that others use with the autistic children is not very difficult. Although this is an important finding, it has not led in any simple way to evidence that it is possible, using the same methods, to rapidly increase spontaneous social interaction initiated by the autistic children. On the other hand, behaviors that are precursors to interaction do seem to change in a more reliable and predictable fashion; these include autistic children's proximity to other people, the amount of time they spend watching other people, and their responsiveness to others' approaches (Lord, 1984; Lord & Hopkins, 1986). These are important steps, particularly for preschool children, in opening opportunities for learning social behaviors.

A number of studies have shown that autistic children can be taught to imitate others with and without objects (Carr & Darcy, 1990; Lovaas, Freitag, Nelson, & Whalen, 1967; Tiegerman & Primavera, 1984). Imitative skills have been shown to generalize to new uses of old objects and to new objects (Carr & Darcy, 1990). Socially directed behaviors, including eye contact, have been shown to increase when a child is being imitated (Dawson & Adams, 1984).

Other specific social skills have also been shown to increase in response to standard behavioral programs (Lovaas *et al.,* 1967), in response to selection of tasks that are more developmentally appropriate (Dawson & Galpert, 1986; Schopler, 1976) and with added structure and increased intrusiveness on the part of the person interacting with the child (Clark & Rutter, 1981; Schopler, 1989). Because many social skills have been shown to improve in situations where demands are at an appropriate developmental level, the use of formal behavioral methods to teach behaviors such as eye contact has often been replaced by more general strategies, including emphasis on communication and structure, and more general social goals (Howlin & Rutter, 1987; Schopler *et al.,* 1990).

Improving Relationships, Affect, and Affectionate Behavior

As with eye contact, behavioral programs have been able to show increases in positive affect and affectionate approaches in children taught specific "affectionate activities" (Lovaas, *et al.,* 1966; McEvoy *et al.,* 1988). However, the general trend has been to work to improve relationships and increase positive affect, in most cases with parents and/or teachers, and then assume that along with changes in the general relationship would come affection, rather than to target individual social behaviors in isolation. Strategies for improving relationships have included decreasing behavior problems, increasing predictability, and maintaining positive attitudes, as well as providing support and information to parents or teachers (Rogers & Lewis, 1989; Schopler, 1989). Social skills programs exist for young, normally developing children in which recognition of emotions and discussions of empathy and ways of expressing emotions take place (Spivack & Shure, 1974). For most autistic children, however, these programs are too difficult and too verbally oriented. Clinical experience suggests that the most easily taught aspect of "appropriate affect" may be helping children label with words or gestures or use objects to show how they would like help; in many cases, this may help to avoid a tantrum or other expression of fear or frustration. Many children can learn to label facial expressions, and in the long run, this may be a useful step toward self-awareness and attention to others' feelings, but for very young children, it is often a skill without much generalization, unless specific efforts are made to tie the labeling to a change in behavior.

Increasing Appropriate Play and Adaptive Skills

Increases in functional, symbolic, and any sort of interactional play have been one of the surprisingly strong results of a number of preschool/school peer-intervention studies (Lord, 1984; Rogers & Lewis, 1989). Even though other aspects of social behaviors seem so context-bound that generalization, if it occurs, has been difficult to document, autistic children can learn to play with objects more like other children. They also seem to be able to transfer this learning to new situations and new partners (Carr & Darcy, 1990). For parents and teachers who are overwhelmed with the number of social skills that autistic children need to be taught, and with the limited generalization often seen outside the classroom or with anyone who is not the parent or teacher, the area of play seems a worthwhile target. Like changes in proximity and attentiveness, play is an important step in becoming more sociable that seems to generalize more easily than other behaviors.

Adaptive skills, such as toileting, dressing, and eating are also often areas of concern for parents. Gains in these areas are one of the most important benefits of parent-as-cotherapist treatment models (Schopler, 1989). There is not sufficient space here to discuss programs in these areas in detail, but more information is available in Sulzer-Azroff and Mayer (1977) regarding toileting and Schopler, Lansing, and Waters (1983) regarding a variety of adaptive activities.

Summary of Treatment Goals

Table 4-2 provides a summary of social treatment goals appropriate for preschool children with autism. This list is loosely adapted from Donnellan and Kilman (1986) and Lord (1990), and is intended to indicate the range of skills and activities that fall in this domain. These are generally, but not strictly, placed in order of presumed difficulty; it is not intended as a hierarchical list in which one skill is required before another can be attained. Not listed because they are covered elsewhere, but also important, are goals of reducing behavior problems and improving communication (see Prizant & Wetherby, this volume; Van Bourgondien, this volume).

General Issues in Treatment

The purpose of this final section is to summarize issues in treatment that have emerged in earlier discussions. As shown in Table 4-3,

Table 4-2. Goals for Social Interventions with Young Autistic Children

Spontaneous and comfortable maintenance of proximity
Imitation and social responsiveness
Functional and beginning symbolic play
Shared activities and cooperation at a simple level
Adaptive skills
Turn-taking
Making initiations
Asking for help and information
Negotiating for space and activities
Alertness to social contexts and appropriate behaviors
Understanding and appropriately expressing affect

Table 4-3. Principles in Providing Treatment
of Social Deficits to Young Autistic Children

Importance of structure and predictability
Active engagement of therapist or teacher
Opportunity for active engagement of child
Involvement of parents
Inseparability of cognition, affect, and social development
Individualization of goals and techniques
Working within a natural environment

six principles underlying effective interventions are proposed. First is the issue of structure and predictability. This includes setting up routines that allow a child to foresee beginnings and ends of social activities, timing of demands, breaks and rewards, and likely behaviors of other people (Donnellan & Kilman, 1986; Lord, 1984). With structure, it is much more likely the child will stay nearby and come to people voluntarily: two critical aspects in any intervention. The second and third principles involve the active engagement of both the person working with the child and the child herself or himself. Research has shown that, if the task is developmentally appropriate, the more actively engaged the teacher or parent or other child is in working with the child, the more socially responsive the child will be (Clark & Rutter, 1981; Lord & Hopkins, 1986). Similarly, the autistic child must be an active participant in the interaction. If he or she remains very passive and has to be prompted throughout an entire activity, the activity may be too difficult or inappropriate for some other reason. It is worthwhile looking for an alternative task that requires less constant direction from the other participant. This is not to say that autistic children should never be taught an activity that requires shaping or prompting, but the goal should be to design interventions in which the child fairly rapidly directs his or her own behavior through a gradually increasing hierarchy of complexity.

A fourth principle is the involvement of parents in all phases of the intervention, if they wish. It is also important to remember that parent–child interaction is a two-way proposition. The child may have affected the parents' ways of interacting just as much as they have affected his or hers. Helping parents modify their behaviors to fit the needs of an autistic child will only be successful if parents are comfortable with what they are expected to do and if it is positive for them. As we try to increase positive affect in the autistic child, we need to recognize as well how his or her parents are feeling.

A fifth principle is to work within everyday environments and to use natural aspects of social situations as much as possible. Similarly, a sixth principle is the importance of recognizing that cognition, affect and social development are inseparably linked and that goals and intervention strategies must always take into account a child's level and motivation in each of these areas. This leads us to the seventh principle, the need for individualization of goals and treatment techniques. The incredible variation in skills and behaviors among autistic children and across social situations must be taken into account.

Finally, questions remain that are not yet answerable, but deserve mention. One is the effect of the age of initiating treatment. It has been generally believed, and was recently suggested in association with a major research project, that the earlier intervention begins, the more it will accomplish (Lovaas, 1987). While it is difficult to argue with this statement, it seems important to consider it on two levels. First, intervention with very young children requires that children be identified as autistic at very young ages (that is, under age 3 years), and it is not clear that this is a reliable judgment, or if it is, how it should be made. Second is the question of what constitutes the most appropriate type of interaction and intervention for very young autistic children (assuming they can be identified reliably). Most models have assumed more is better: that is, that more treatment hours, more teachers, more goals will result in greater improvement; however, this may not be the case, particularly when the demands on families_(particularly mothers) are considered. These are important questions that will require very careful work to answer.

Another issue is the length of time taken to acquire some social goals, particularly those taught in formal behavioral paradigms (Lovaas et al., 1973; Taras, Matson, & Leary, 1988). If it requires hundreds of trials or hours of intervention or months of work for a child to acquire a simple imitation skill or to make an appropriate approach, then a change in strategy or goal seems warranted. On the other hand, it is always difficult to admit defeat. Similarly, generalization across social behaviors has not been particularly strong, except in play skills, imitation, and in those behaviors that are almost "presocial," that is, those that involve spontaneous watching of other children and voluntarily staying near other people. Perhaps this is as much as we can expect, or perhaps we should be breaking down treatment goals and interventions into even smaller steps.

CONCLUSION

Altogether, the area of social development in very young autistic children is one of great promise. More is learned each day about the nature of and contributing factors to autistic children's social difficulties and about ways to intercede, so that continued opportunities for learning and interaction occur for each child. Let us combine this optimism with careful consideration of realistic goals for individual children and deliberate attention to generalization so that the result is general knowledge that can be used with many children and measurable change in the children with whom we work.

REFERENCES

Acredolo, L., & Goodwyn, S. (1988). Symbolic gesturing in normal infants. *Child Development, 59,* 450–466.
Adrien, J. L., Ornitz, E., Barthelmy, C., Sauvage, D., & LeLord, G. (1987). The presence or absence of certain behaviors associated with infantile autism in severely retarded autistic and nonautistic retarded children and very young normal children. *Journal of Autism and Developmental Disorders, 17,* 407–416.
American Psychiatric Association. (1980). *Diagnostic and statistical manual of mental disorders* (3rd ed.). Washington, DC: Author.
American Psychiatric Association. (1987). *Diagnostic and statistical manual of mental disorders* (3rd ed., rev.). Washington, DC: Author.
Anderson, S. R., Avery, D. L., DiPietro, E. K., Edwards, G. L., & Christian, W. P. (1987). Intensive home-based early intervention with autistic children. *Education and Treatment of Children, 10,* 352–366.
Attwood, A., Frith, J., & Hermelin, B. (1988). The understanding and use of interpersonal gestures by autistic and Down's syndrome children. *Journal of Autism and Developmental Disorders, 18,* 241–258.
Baltaxe, C. A. M., & Guthrie, D. (1987). The use of primary sentence stress by normal, aphasic, and autistic children. *Journal of Autism and Developmental Disorders, 17,* 255–271.
Baron-Cohen, S. (1988). Social and pragmatic deficits in autism: Cognitive or affective? *Journal of Autism and Developmental Disorders, 18,* 379–402.
Baron-Cohen, S. (1989). Joint-attention deficits in autism: Towards a cognitive analysis. *Development and Psychopathology, 1,* 185–189.
Bartak, L., Rutter, M., & Cox, A. (1975). A comparative study of infantile autism and specific developmental receptive language disorder: I. The children. *British Journal of Psychiatry, 126,* 127–145.
Bebko, J. M., Konstantareas, M. M., & Springer, J. (1987). Parent and professional evaluations of

family stress associated with characteristics of autism. *Journal of Autism and Developmental Disorders, 17*, 565–576.

Brownell, C. A. (1986). Convergent developments: Cognitive-developmental correlates of growth in infant/toddler peer skills. *Child Development, 57*, 275–286.

Carr, E. G. (1983, August). *Application of pragmatics to conceptualization and treatment of severe behavior problems in children.* Paper presented at the Annual Convention of the American Psychological Association, Anaheim, CA.

Carr, E. G., & Darcy, M. (1990). Setting generality of peer modeling in children with autism. *Journal of Autism and Developmental Disorders, 20*, 45–59.

Chess, S., & Rosenberg, M. (1974). Clinical differentiation among children with initial language complaints. *Journal of Autism and Childhood Schizophrenia, 4*, 99–109.

Cicchetti, D., & Serafica, F. C. (1981). Interplay among behavioral systems: Illustrations from the study of attachment, affiliation, and wariness in young children with Down's syndrome. *Developmental Psychology, 17*, 36–49.

Clark, P., & Rutter, M. (1977). Compliance and resistance in autistic children. *Journal of Autism and Childhood Schizophrenia, 1*, 33–48.

Clark, P., & Rutter, M. (1981). Autistic children's responses to structure and to interpersonal demands. *Journal of Autism and Developmental Disorders, 11*, 201–217.

Clarke-Stewart, A. (1978). Recasting the lone stranger. In J. Glick & K. A. Clarke-Stewart (Eds.), *The development of social understanding* (pp. 56–93). New York: Gardiner.

Cohen, D. J., Paul, R., & Volkmar, F. R. (1987). Issues in the classification of pervasive developmental disorders and associated conditions. In D. J. Cohen & A. M. Donnellan (Eds.), *Handbook of autism and pervasive developmental disorders* (pp. 20–40). New York: John Wiley & Sons.

Collis, G. M., & Schaffer, H. R. (1975). Synchronization of visual attention in mother–infant pairs. *Journal of Child Psychology and Psychiatry, 16*, 315–320.

Curcio, F. (1978). Sensorimotor functioning and communication in mute autistic children. *Journal of Autism and Childhood Schizophrenia, 8*, 281–292.

Dahl, E. K., Cohen, D. J., & Provence, S. (1986). Clinical and multivariate approaches to the nosology of pervasive developmental disorders. *Journal of American Academy of Child Psychiatry, 25*, 170–180.

Dahlgren, S. O., & Gillberg, C. (1989). Symptoms in the first two years of life: A preliminary population study of infantile autism. *European Archives of Psychiatric and Neurological Science, 283*, 169–174.

Dawson, G., & Adams, A. (1984). Imitation and social responsiveness in autistic children. *Journal of Abnormal Child Psychology, 12*, 209–226.

Dawson, G., & Galpert, L. (1986). A developmental model for facilitating the social behavior of autistic children. In E. Schopler & G. B. Mesibov (Eds.), *Social behavior in autism* (pp. 237–261). New York: Plenum Press.

Dawson, G., Hill, D., Spencer, A., Galpert, L., & Watson, L. (1990). Affective exchanges between young autistic children and their mothers. *Journal of Abnormal Child Psychology, 18*, 335–345.

Dawson, G., & Lewy, A. (1989). Arousal, attention, and the socioemotional impairments of individuals with autism. In G. Dawson (Ed.), *Autism: Nature, diagnosis, and treatment* (pp. 49–74). New York: Guilford Press.

Dawson, G., & McKissick, F. C. (1984). Self-recognition in autistic children. *Journal of Autism and Developmental Psychology, 14*, 383–394.

DeMyer, M. K., Alpern, G. D., Barton, S., DeMyer, W. E., Churchill, D. W., Hingtgen, J. N., Bryson, C. Q., Pontius, W., & Kimberlin, C. (1972). Imitation in autistic, early schizophrenic, and nonpsychotic subnormal children. *Journal of Autism and Childhood Schizophrenia,* *2*, 264–287.

DeMyer, M. K., Mann, N. A., Tilton, J. R., & Loew, L. H. (1967). Toy–play behavior and use of body by autistic and normal children as reported by mothers. *Psychological Reports, 21,* 973–981.

Donnellan, A. M., & Kilman, B. A. (1986). Behavioral approaches to social skill development in autism: Strengths, misapplications, and alternatives. In E. Schopler & G. B. Mesibov (Eds.), *Social behavior in autism* (pp. 213–236). New York: Plenum Press.

Dunn, J. (1988). Sibling influences on childhood development. *Journal of Child Psychology and Psychiatry, 29,* 119–128.

Dyer, K., & Peck, C. A. (1987). Current perspectives on social/communication curricula for students with autism and severe handicaps. *Education and Treatment of Children, 10,* 338–351.

Ferrari, M., & Matthews, W. (1983). Self-recognition deficits in autism: Syndrome-specific or general developmental delay? *Journal of Autism and Developmental Disorders, 13,* 317–324.

Frith, U. (1989). *Autism: Explaining the enigma.* Oxford: Blackwell Press.

Gillberg, C., Ehlers, S., Schaumann, H., Jakobsson, G., Dahlgren, S. O., Lindblom, R., Bagenholm, A., Tjuus, T., & Blidner, E. (1990). Autism under age three years. A clinical study of 28 cases referred for autistic symptoms in infancy. *Journal of Child Psychology and Psychiatry, 31,* 921–934.

Harris, P. L. (1989). The autistic child's impaired conception of mental states. *Developmental and psychopathology, 1,* 191–195.

Harris, S. L., Handleman, J. S., Kristoff, B., Bass, L., & Gordon, R. (1990). Changes in language development among autistic and peer children in segregated and integrated preschool settings. *Journal of Autism and Developmental Disorders, 20,* 23–31.

Hermelin, B., & O'Connor, N. (1970). *Psychological experiments with autistic children.* Oxford: Pergamon Press.

Hetherington, E. M. (1983). Volume IV: Socialization, personality, and social development. In P. H. Mussen (Ed.), *Handbook of child psychology* (4th ed.). New York: Wiley.

Hobson, R. P. (1986). The autistic child's appraisal of expressions of emotion. *Journal of Child Psychology and Psychiatry, 27,* 321–342.

Hobson, R. P. (1991). Methodological issues for experiments on autistic individuals' perception and understanding of emotion. *Journal of Child Psychology and Psychiatry, 32,* 1135–1138.

Hobson, R. P. (in press). Understanding persons: The role of affect. In S. Baron-Cohen, H. Tager-Flusberg & P. Cohen (Eds.). *Understanding other minds: Perspectives in autism.* Oxford: Oxford University Press.

Hobson, R. P., Ouston, J., & Lee, A. (1989). Naming emotion in faces and voices: Abilities and disabilities in autism and mental retardation. *British Journal of Developmental Psychology, 7,* 237–250.

Howes, C. (1987). Peer interaction of young children. *Monographs of the Society for Research in Child Development, 53* (1).

Howlin, P. Cantwell, D., Marchant, R., Berger, M., & Rutter, M. (1973). Analyzing mothers' speech to young autistic children: A methodological study. *Journal of Abnormal Child Psychology, 1,* 317–339.

Howlin, P., & Rutter, M. (187). *Treatment of autistic children.* Chichester: Wiley.

Hoyson, M., Jamison, B., & Strain, P. S. (1984). Individualized group instruction of normally developing and autistic-like children: The LEAP curriculum model. *Journal of the Division for Early Childhood, 8,* 157–172.

Jacobson, J. W., & Ackerman, L. J. (1990). Differences in adaptive functioning among people with autism or mental retardation. *Journal of Autism and Developmental Disorders, 20,* 205–220.

Kanner, L. (1943). Autistic disturbances of affective contact. *Nervous Child, 2,* 217–250.

Kasari, C., Sigman, M., Mundy, P., & Yirmiya, N. (1988). Caregiver interactions with autistic children. *Journal of Abnormal Child Psychology, 16,* 45–56.

Kasari, C., Sigman, M., Mundy, P., & Yirmiya, N. (1990). Affective sharing in the context of joint attention interactions of normal, autistic, and mentally retarded children. *Journal of Autism and Developmental Disorders, 20,* 87–100.

Knobloch, H., & Pasamanick, B. (1975). Some etiologic and prognostic factors in early infantile autism and psychosis. *Pediatrics, 55,* 182–191.

Koegel, R. L., Schreibman, L., Britten, K. R., Burke, J. C., & O'Neill, R. E. (1982). A comparison of parent training to direct clinic treatment. In R. L. Koegel, A. Rincover, & A. L. Egel (Eds.), *Educating and understanding autistic children.* San Diego: College Hill Press.

Konstantareas, M. M., & Homatidis, S. (1989). Assessing child symptom severity and stress in parents of autistic children. *Journal of Child Psychology and Psychiatry, 30,* 459–470.

Kubicek L. F. (1980). Organization in two mother–infant interactions involving a normal infant and his fraternal twin who was later diagnosed as autistic. In T. M. Field, S. Goldberg, D. Stern, & A. M. Sostek (Eds.), *High-risk infants and children: Adult and peer interactions* (pp. 99–110). New York: Academic Press.

Lamb, M. (1977). The development of mother–infant and father–infant attachments in the second year of life. *Developmental Psychology, 13,* 639–649.

Le Couteur, A., Rutter, M., Lord, C., Rios, P., Robertson, S., Holdgrafer, M., & McLennan, J. D. (1989). Autism Diagnostic Interview: A standardized investigator-based instrument. *Journal of Autism and Developmental Disorders, 19,* 363–387.

Leslie, A. M. (1987). Pretense and representation: The origins of "Theory of mind." *Psychological Review, 94,* 412–426.

Levine, J. M., & Demb, H. B. (1987). Characteristics of preschool children diagnosed as having an atypical pervasive developmental disorder. *Developmental and Behavioral Pediatrics, 8,* 77–82.

Lewis, M. (1987). Social development in infancy and early childhood. In J. D. Osofsky (Ed.), *Handbook of infant development* (pp. 579–647). New York: John Wiley & Sons.

Lord, C. (1984). The development of peer relations in children with autism. In F. J. Morrison, C. Lord, & D. P. Keating (Eds.), *Advances in applied developmental psychology* (pp. 165–229). New York: Academic Press.

Lord, C. (1985). Autism and the comprehension of language. In E. Schopler & G. B. Mesibov (Eds.) *Communication problems in autism* (pp. 257–281). New York: Plenum Press.

Lord, C. (1990). A cognitive behavioral model for the treatment of social-communicative deficits in adolescents in autism. In R. McMahon & R. Peters (Eds.), *Behavior disorders of adolescence: Research, intervention, and policy in clinical and school settings* (pp. 155–174). New York: Plenum Press.

Lord, C., & Hopkins, J. M. (1986). The social behavior of autistic children with younger and same-age nonhandicapped peers. *Journal of Autism and Developmental Disorders, 16,* 249–262.

Lord, C., & Magill, J. (1989). Methodological and theoretical issues in studying peer-directed behavior and autism. In G. Dawson (Ed.), *Autism: Nature, diagnosis, and treatment* (pp. 326–345). New York: Guilford Press.

Lord, C., Merrin, D. J., Vest, L., & Kelly, K. M. (1983). Communicative behavior of adults with an autistic four-year-old boy and his nonhandicapped twin brother. *Journal of Autism and Developmental Disorders, 13,* 1–17.

Lord, C., Rutter, M., Goode, S., Heemsbergen, J., Jordan, H., Mawhood, L. (1989). Autism diagnostic observation schedule: A standardized observation of communicative and social behavior. *Journal of Autism and Developmental Disorders, 19,* 185–212.

Lovaas, O. I. (1987). Behavioral treatment and normal educational and intellectual functioning in young autistic children. *Journal of Consulting and Clinical Psychology, 55,* 3–9.

Lovaas, O. I., Freitag, G., Kinder, M. I., Rubenstein, B. D., Schaeffer, B., & Simmons, J. Q. (1966). Establishment of social reinforcers in two schizophrenic children on the basis of food. *Journal of Experimental Child Psychology, 4,* 109–125.

Lovaas, O. I., Freitag, G., Nelson, K., & Whalen, C. (1967). The establishment of imitation and its use for the development of complex behavior in schizophrenic children. *Behaviour Research and Therapy, 5,* 171–181.

Lovaas, O. I., Koegel, R., Simmons, J. Q., & Long, J. S. (1973). Some generalization and follow-up measures on autistic children in behavior therapy. *Journal of Applied Behavior Analysis, 6,* 131–166.

Loveland, K., & Landry, S. (1986). Joint attention and language in autism and developmental language delay. *Journal of Autism and Developmental Disorders, 16,* 335–349.

Massie, H. N., & Rosenthal, J. (1984). *Childhood psychosis in the first four years of life.* New York: McGraw-Hill.

McEvoy, M. A., Nordquist, V. M., Twardosz, S., Heckaman, K. A., Wehby, J. H., & Denny, R. K. (1988). Promoting autistic children's peer interactions in an integrated early childhood setting using affection activities. *Journal of Applied Behavior Analysis, 21,* 193–200.

McHale, S. M., & Gamble, W. C. (1986). Mainstreaming handicapped children in public school settings: Challenges and limitations. In E. Schopler and G. B. Mesibov (Eds.), *Social behavior in autism* (pp. 191–212). New York: Plenum Press.

McHale, S. M., Olley, J. G., & Marcus, L. M. (1981, April). *Variations across settings in autistic children's play.* Paper presented at biannual meetings of the Society for Research in Child Development, Boston, MA.

Mundy, P., Sigman, M., Ungerer, J., & Sherman, T. (1986). Defining the social deficits of autism: The contribution of nonverbal communication measures. *Journal of Child Psychology and Psychiatry, 27,* 657–669.

Neuman, C., & Hill, S. (1978). Self-recognition and stimulus preference in autistic children. *Developmental Psychobiology, 11,* 571–578.

O'Neill, P. J., & Lord, C. (1982). Functional and semantic characteristics of child-directed speech of autistic children. In D. Park (Ed.), *Proceedings from the International Meetings for the National Society for Autistic Children* (pp. 79–82). Washington, DC: National Society for Autistic Children.

Odom, S. L., & Strain, P. S. (1986). Comparison of peer-initiation and teacher-antecedent interventions for promoting reciprocal social interaction of autistic preschoolers. *Journal of Applied Behavior Analysis, 19,* 59–71.

Ohta, M., Nagai, Y., Hara, H., & Sasaki, M. (1987). Parental perception of behavioral symptoms in Japanese autistic children. *Journal of Autism and Developmental Disorders, 17,* 549–564.

Ornitz, E. M., Guthrie, D., & Farley, A. H. (1977). The early development of autistic children. *Journal of Autism and Childhood Schizophrenia, 7,* 207–229.

Park, C. C. (1986). Social growth in autism: A parent's perspective. In E. Schopler & G. B. Mesibov (Eds.), *Social behavior in autism* (pp. 81–99). New York: Plenum Press.

Parke, R. D., & Tinsley, B. J. (1987). Family interaction in infancy. In J. D. Osofsky (Ed.), *Handbook of infant development* (pp. 579–647). New York: John Wiley & Sons.

Podrouzek, W., & Furrow, D. (1988). Preschoolers' use of eye contact while speaking: The influence of sex, age, and conversational partner. *Journal of Psycholinguistic Research, 17,* 89–98.

Prizant, B. M., & Wetherby, A. M. (in press). Communication in preschool autistic children. In E. Schopler, M. E. Van Bourgondien, & M. Bristol (Eds.), *Preschool issues in autism and related developmental handicaps.* New York: Plenum Press.

Rescorla, L. (1988). Cluster analytic identification of autistic preschoolers. *Journal of Autism and Developmental Disorders, 18*, 475–492.

Ricks, D. M., & Wing, L. (1976). Language, communication, and use of symbols. In L. Wing (Ed.), *Early childhood autism* (pp. 93–134). Oxford: Pergamon Press.

Rogers, S. J., & Lewis, H. (1989). An effective day treatment model for young children with pervasive developmental disorders. *Journal of the American Academy of Child and Adolescent Psychiatry, 28*, 207–214.

Rumsey, J. M., Rapoport, M. D., & Sceery, W. R. (1985). Autistic children as adults: Psychiatric, social, and behavioral outcomes. *Journal of the American Academy of Child Psychiatry, 24*, 465–473.

Rutter, M. (1985). Infantile autism. In D. Shaffer, A. Erhardt, & L. Greenhill (Eds.). *A clinician's guide to child psychiatry* (pp. 48–78). New York: Free Press.

Rutter, M., Le Couteur, A., Lord, C. (in press). Brief report: Autism diagnostic interview–revised. *Journal of Autism and Developmental Disorders.*

Schopler, E. (1976). Towards reducing behavior problems in autistic children. In L. Wing (Ed.), *Early childhood autism* (pp. 221–246). London: Pergamon Press.

Schopler, E. (1989). Principles for directing both educational treatment and research. In C. Gillberg (Ed.), *Diagnosis and treatment of autism* (pp. 167–183). New York: Plenum Press.

Schopler, E., Lansing, M., & Waters, L. (1983). *Teaching activities for autistic children (Vol. 3)* Austin, TX: Pro-Ed.

Schopler, E., & Reichler, R. J. (1972). How well do parents understand their own psychotic child? *Journal of Autism and Childhood Schizophrenia, 2*, 387–400.

Schopler, E., Reichler, R. J., Bashford, A., Lansing, M. D., & Marcus, L. M. (1990). *Psychoeducational profile revised.* Austin, TX: Pro-Ed.

Schopler, E., Reichler, R. J., & Renner, B. R. (1986) *The Childhood Autism Rating Scale (CARS).* Los Angeles: Western Psychological.

Schreibman, L. (1988). Parent training as a means of facilitating generalization in autistic children. In R. H. Horner, G. Dunlap, & R. L. Koegel (Eds.), *Generalization and maintenance: Lifestyle changes in applied settings.* New York: Pergamon.

Shapiro, T., Frosch, E., & Arnold, S. (1987). Communicative interaction between mothers and their autistic children: Application of a new instrument and changes after treatment. *Journal of the American Academy of Child Psychiatry, 26*, 485–590.

Shapiro, T., Sherman, M., Calamari, G., & Koch, D. (1987). Attachment in autism and other developmental disorders. *Journal of the American Academy of Child Psychiatry, 26*, 480–484.

Sherman, J., Barker, P., Lorimer, P., Swinson, R., & Factor, D. C. (1988). Treatment of autistic children: Relative effectiveness of residential, out-patient, and home-based interventions. *Child Psychiatry and Human Development, 19*, 109–125.

Sherman, M., Shapiro, J., & Glassman, M. (1983). Play and language in developmentally disordered preschoolers: A new approach to classification. *Journal of the American Academy of Child Psychiatry, 22*, 511–524.

Sigman, M., & Mundy, P. (1989). Social attachments in autistic children. *American Academy of Child and Adolescent Psychiatry, 28*, 74–81.

Sigman, M., Mundy, P., Sherman, T., & Ungerer, J. (1986). Social interactions of autistic, mentally retarded, and normal children and their caregivers. *Journal of Child Psychology and Psychiatry, 27*, 647–656.

Sigman, M., & Ungerer, J. (1984). Attachment behaviors in autistic children. *Journal of Autism and Developmental Disorders, 14*, 231–244.

Snow, M., Hertzig, M., & Shapiro, T. (1987). Expression of emotion in young autistic children. *Journal of the American Academy of Child and Adolescent Psychiatry, 26*, 836–838.

Sparrow, S., Balla, D., & Cicchetti, D. (1984). *Vineland adaptive behavior scales.* Circle Pines, MN: American Guidance Service.

Spiker, D., & Ricks, M. (1983). Visual self recognition in autistic children: Developmental relationships. *Child Development, 55,* 214–225.

Spivak, G., & Shure, M. B. (1974). *Social adjustment in young children.* San Francisco: Jossey-Bass.

Stone, W. L., & Lemanak, K. L. (1990). Parental report of social behaviors in autistic preschoolers. *Journal of Autism and Developmental Disorders, 20,* 513–522.

Stone, W. L., Lemanak, K. L., Fishel, P. T., Fernandez, M. C., & Altemeier, W. A. (1990). Play and imitation skills in the diagnosis of young autistic children. *Pediatrics, 86,* 267–272.

Strain, P. S., & Cooke, T. P. (1976). An observational investigation of two elementary-age autistic children during free play. *Psychology in the Schools, 13,* 82–91.

Sulzer-Azroff, B., & Mayer, G. R. (1977). *Applying behavior analysis procedures with children and youth.* New York: Holt, Rinehart, & Winston.

Taras, M. E., Matson, J. L., & Leary, C. (1988). Training social interpersonal skills in two autistic children. *Journal of Behavior Therapy and Experimental Psychiatry, 19,* 275–280.

Tiegerman, E., & Primavera, L. H. (1984). Imitating the autistic child: Facilitating communicative gaze behavior. *Journal of Autism and Developmental Disorders, 14,* 27–38.

Ungerer, J. A., & Sigman, M. (1981). Symbolic play and language comprehension in autistic children. *Journal of the American Academy of Child Psychiatry, 20,* 318–337.

Van Berckelaer-Onnes, I. A. (1983). *Early childhood autism: A child-rearing problem.* Lisse, The Netherlands: Swets & Zeitlinger.

Volkmar, F. R. (1987). Diagnostic issues in the pervasive developmental disorders. *Journal of Child Psychology and Psychiatry, 28,* 365–369.

Volkmar, F. R., & Cohen, D. J. (1988). Neurobiologic aspects of autism. *The New England Journal of Medicine, 318,* 1390–1392.

Volkmar, F. R., Sparrow, S. S., Goudreau, D., Cicchetti, D. V., Paul, R., & Cohen, D. J. (1987). Social deficits in autism: An operational approach using the Vineland Adaptive Behavior Scales. *Journal of the American Academy of Child and Adolescent Psychiatry, 26,* 156–161.

Watson, L., & Marcus, L. M. (1988). Diagnosis and assessment of preschool children. In E. Schopler & G. Mesibov (Eds.), *Diagnosis and Assessment in Autism* (pp. 271–301). New York: Plenum Press.

Weeks, S. J., & Hobson, R. P. (1987). The salience of facial expression for autistic children. *Journal of Child Psychology and Psychiatry, 28,* 137–152.

Wenar, C., Ruttenberg, R. A., Kalish-Weiss, B., & Wolf, E. G. (1986). The development of normal and autistic children: A comparative study. *Journal of Autism and Developmental Disorders, 16,* 317–334.

Wetherby, A. M., & Prutting, C. A. (1984). Profiles of communicative and cognitive–social abilities in autistic children. *Journal of Speech and Hearing Research, 27,* 364–377.

Wing, L. (1976). Diagnosis, clinical description, and prognosis. In L. Wing (Ed.), *Early childhood autism* (pp. 15–64). London: Pergamon Press.

Yirmiya, N., Kasari, C., Sigman, M., & Mundy, P. (1989). Facial expressions of affect in autistic, mentally retarded, and normal children. *Journal of Child Psychology and Psychiatry, 30,* 725–736.

5

Communication in Preschool Autistic Children

BARRY M. PRIZANT and AMY M. WETHERBY

COMMUNICATION IN PRESCHOOL AUTISTIC CHILDREN

Over the past decade, major advances have been made in understanding communication and social problems of young children with autism. This progress has resulted in a greater emphasis on specific communicative symptomatology in diagnostic criteria for autistic disorder (American Psychiatric Association, 1987). Thus, communication characteristics in autism are now considered to be central to our understanding of the syndrome, and to assessment and treatment efforts. This increased emphasis on language and communication in both theory and practice has been fueled by a confluence of knowledge from a variety of orientations (Prizant & Wetherby, 1989). Whereas approaches to assessing and enhancing communication in the 1960s and 1970s relied primarily upon behavioral models of speech training (e.g., Lovaas, 1977; 1981), developmental and pragmatic approaches have had an increasing influence since the late 1970s. Earlier behavioral approaches demonstrated that children with autism can learn specific skills in vocal and motor imitation, word production, and word discrimination. How-

BARRY M. PRIZANT • Division of Communication Disorders, Emerson College, Boston, Massachusetts 02116   AMY M. WETHERBY • Department of Communication Disorders, Florida State University, Tallahassee, Florida 32306.

Preschool Issues in Autism, edited by Eric Schopler *et al.* Plenum Press, New York, 1993.

ever, true progress in social-communicative competence (i.e., development of spontaneous verbal and nonverbal communication) was often
of limited interest to clinicians and researchers of a more traditional
behavioral orientation (Bryen & Joyce, 1985; Prizant, 1982; Prizant &
Wetherby, 1989), and thus was rarely measured and/or reported.

It has been argued that a rigid adherence to training skills following a developmental sequence, which has mistakenly been equated to a
developmental approach, may be of questionable value with persons
with severe handicaps including autism. We have argued that training to
a developmental checklist, or "readiness approaches," should not be
confused with an approach to communication enhancement grounded in
our knowledge of communication in development of children without
disabilities (Prizant & Wetherby, 1989). Bruner (1983), one of the fore-
most developmental psychologists of the past half-century, noted that a
developmental approach *does not* dictate that so-called specific pre-
requisites must be acquired prior to the acquisition of more advanced
skills or knowledge. Rather, a child's ability to acquire a certain level
of knowledge or certain skills will be framed by his/her developmental capacities across various domains. In other words, developmental
principles should guide, but not dictate, assessment and intervention
practices. Preschool children with autism would seem to be excellent
candidates for approaches that rely upon guidelines derived from developmental processes and content. Experienced clinicians and caregivers have known for years the ability of many autistic children to be
"trained" to acquire seemingly advanced skills (e.g., sentence repetition in the absence of comprehension; decoding of written language
in the absence of comprehension). Such skills may present a spuri-
ous picture of progress, and encourage ill-informed intervention efforts
when overall developmental capacities and usefulness of such skills are
not considered.

In this chapter, we will review current knowledge regarding the
contribution of early social-communicative patterns to early detection of
autism, and approaches to communication assessment and enhancement
for preschool children with autism and related social-communicative
disorders. The impact of developmental literature will be highlighted
throughout. Particular emphasis will be placed on the uneven developmental profile observed in autism, especially in social-communicative
development, which has a profound impact on early differential diagno-

sis, communication assessment, and communication enhancement. Emphasis also will be placed on how developmental information provides a framework for communication assessment and enhancement, and on the role of caregivers and the family as central partners in the process of helping young children with autism reach their social-communicative potential.

Review of Early Symptomatology and Early Developmental Patterns in Communication

Most children identified as having the autistic syndrome are reported by their caregivers to demonstrate symptoms within the first two years of life (Short & Schopler, 1988). However, in practice, these children may not be diagnosed until three to five years of age at the earliest, and many are diagnosed at a later age. Identification and diagnosis of autism by professionals during the first 18 months of life is an extremely rare occurrence. Factors precluding early detection include the variability of behavior in very young children (normally developing, at-risk, or disabled), lack of appropriate referrals by professionals to whom parents expressed concern, and/or the family's lack of knowledge of services or access to services.

Research findings based on parental retrospective accounts suggest that there may not be a single early behavioral profile characterizing children later diagnosed as autistic. Coleman and Gillberg (1985) discussed two general "modes of presentation": the "model" baby who presents few demands, may be lethargic, and appears to want to be left alone; and the "terrible" or highly irritable baby who may have sleeping problems, frequently screams or cries, and may be difficult to console. Furthermore, there may be at least two different subtypes of autistic children distinguished on the basis of clinical onset (Freeman & Ritvo, 1984). As many as 80% to 90% of children diagnosed as autistic have a history of developmental delays and observable symptoms early in life, with the remainder having a history of normal development in the first year or two of life with subsequent developmental arrests or regression accompanied by the onset of specific symptoms.

Early symptomatology in children with onset in the first year includes specific aspects of early social and communicative functioning, as well as nonspecific symptomatology, which may be only indirectly related to the core problems of social and communication deficits in autism (e.g., hyperactivity, stereotyped motor patterns, sleep disturbances). Specific symptomatology related to the social and communication impairments in young autistic children may include absence of social reciprocity through action and vocalization prior to one year, limited social orientation, absence of conventional nonverbal communication (e.g., pointing, requesting, showing gestures, head shakes and nods), and gaze aversion. Beyond two years of age, absence of speech in approximately 50% of young autistic children, and delayed development of speech in children who eventually do speak may cause concern to caregivers. In as many as 85% of children with autism who develop speech, immediate and delayed echolalia (i.e., the immediate or delayed repetition of speech produced by others) is characteristic of early speech patterns (Prizant, 1987; Schuler & Prizant, 1985), which may represent a "gestalt" or chunking strategy for acquiring language (i.e., a rote memorization strategy rather than semantic-based strategy) (Prizant, 1983). Some children who develop speech may experience "speech loss." Kurita (1985) reported that 37.2% of a sample of 261 Japanese children lost meaningful speech prior to 30 months of age. In addition to obvious problems in expressive communication and expressive language, difficulties in language comprehension are pervasive, and social and symbolic play may be strikingly limited or absent in early development (Sigman, Ungerer, Mundy, & Sherman, 1987). Social interactions may have a one-sided quality, with adults or other children having to take the major responsibility for initiating and maintaining contact.

Most researchers now agree that for a child to be diagnosed as having Autistic Disorder, a subcategory of Pervasive Developmental Disorder in the current *DSM-III-R* (APA, 1987), symptomatology must be documented in areas of verbal and nonverbal communication, social-affective competence, and language related cognitive abilities (e.g., symbolic play, imitation). Interestingly, these critical dimensions of the impairment in autism are closely related to what Stern (1985) has implicated as the three major dimensions of a child's emotional development and development of a sense of self. These include the sharing of attention, or interattentionality, the sharing of intention or interintentionality, and the sharing of affect, or interaffectivity. Competencies in joint attention, joint activity, expression of communicative intent, and affective signaling emerge within the first year of life in normally developing children, and provide the underpinnings of competence in later emerging social, affective, and communicative behavior (Bruner, 1981; Bates, O'Connell, & Shore, 1987; Prizant and Wetherby, 1990). Thus, it may be that many young children with autism have a limited foundation for underpinnings of development that may be central to social/emotional and social-communicative growth.

This is not to say that young children with autism are *incapable* of making significant strides in these areas of development. In fact, reports of outcomes of children with autism who received early intervention services are encouraging (Lovaas, 1987; Fenske, Zalenski, Krantz, & McClannahan, 1985; Powers, 1992). It is our contention that with early identification and early intervention initiatives driven by full implementation of Public Law 99-457, more successful outcomes for children with autism who receive early intervention services will continue to be reported.

In early intervention and preschool services, greater emphasis is being placed on early communication and social-affective competence as the central focus in working with young children with autistic symptoms and their families (Prizant & Wetherby, 1988). Early communication intervention also may serve as an approach to secondary prevention of later socioemotional limitations and behavioral problems (Prizant & Wetherby, 1988; Prizant & Meyer, in press), as advances in communication have been shown to be inversely correlated with behavioral problems and disruptive behavior (Carr & Durand, 1985).

Developmental and Functional Considerations in Providing Services to Preschool Children with Autism

In recent years, clinicians and educators have been debating the question of how goals and objectives for young children with autism and related disabilities should be derived. On one extreme are those who focus primarily on the functional needs of a child relative to his or her chronological age (Brown, Branston, Hamre-Nietupski, Pumpian, Certo, & Gruenewald, 1979), with minimal emphasis placed on potential contributions from literature on normal language and communication development. On the other hand, developmentally oriented clinicians, especially those with expertise in language and communication development, have tended to focus on approaches that attempt to move children along a developmental track based upon research on language and communication development (Lahey, 1988). We have argued elsewhere (Prizant & Wetherby, 1989) that so-called functional approaches (which tend to be behaviorally-oriented) and developmental approaches need not be viewed as mutually exclusive. That is, for communication enhancement activities to be most relevant for young children with autism and their families, approaches must be guided by both a child's developmental capacities in communication and social-cognitive abilities, as well as by the child's and family's immediate and future needs. These needs may include increasing functional skills to enhance independence in the child, and reducing stress on the family by providing appropriate tangible and psychosocial supports. Furthermore, the unique learning style and patterns of abilities and disabilities in autism must be taken into consideration. In our experience, however, many educators and clinicians tend to lean heavily towards either developmental approaches or functional/behavioral approaches, to the virtual exclusion of integrating the best practices from both approaches.

In order to address issues raised by both orientations, communication assessment and enhancement will be discussed relative to contributions of the developmental literature to the content of both assessment and enhancement efforts. Functional considerations will focus primarily on child and family needs based on the child's chronological age, and age appropriate contexts and activities for communication assessment and enhancement. Issues in early communication enhancement that require special consideration will also be presented.

COMMUNICATION ASSESSMENT

It is our belief that communication assessment should not be undertaken with the *sole* purpose of differential diagnosis. That is, assessment efforts should always be considered the first, and possibly one of the most crucial steps toward planning for communication enhancement (Prizant & Wetherby, 1993). However, the value of accurate assessment for differential diagnosis of preschool children should not be underestimated. This is especially true for children with autistic symptoms, due to the degree of stress families experience based on the ambiguity of the syndrome, the confusion caused by multiple diagnoses exacerbated by possible disagreement among professionals, and the lack of concrete explanations for the difficulties observed (Bristol, 1985). The communication assessment also is one of the most important assessments for differential diagnosis. As noted, the most widely used current diagnostic scheme for autism (i.e., Autistic Disorder; APA, 1987) highlights symptomatology in communicative, social, and symbolic functioning. Furthermore, it is not just delays in communication and language development, as much as the *quality* of communicative and social impairments that differentiate children with autism from children with other developmental and communication disorders (APA, 1987). Thus, for very young children, clarification of the nature of the disability may help to decrease caregiver stress, and substantiate the need for appropriate educational, clinical and support services for both the child and family (Wetherby & Prizant, 1992).

Contexts of Assessment

Since speech, language and communication impairments in autism are most apparent in the social use of language and communication, traditional formal assessment instruments that focus on form or sophistication of communication, rather than social use of communicative acts, may have limited use (Prizant, 1988; Prizant & Schuler, 1987a). Clinicians and educators, therefore, must rely on systematic use of informal procedures, or more structured procedures approximating natural interactions, to assess communication (Prizant & Wetherby, 1993; Wetherby & Prizant, 1992). Furthermore, preschool children with autism typically are most comfortable and familiar within the interpersonal context of the family, the home environment, or familiar routines and activities. Ideally, communication assessment must take into account children's abilities in familiar and unfamiliar contexts to obtain a representative picture. Assessment of abilities in the home environment may be derived from direct observation in the home, in-depth parental report and interview, and/or systematic observation of the child by caregivers with subsequent sharing of information with clinicians (Prizant & Wetherby, 1985).

Caregivers also should be centrally involved in the assessment process, as separation of preschool children from caregivers for assessment purposes may, in some cases, cause significant stress and anxiety for caregivers and children. The radical change inherent in an unfamiliar environment may add to the stress for some children, resulting in assessment data that could hardly be called representative of a child's communicative behavior in more comfortable and familiar contexts. Thus, communication assessment should include observation of caregiver/child interaction, as well as the use of informal procedures designed to elicit spontaneous communication, where caregivers have the opportunity to observe and comment upon their child's behavior. Information elicited during caregiver interviews may include whether communicative skills have been observed in other environments, clarification of idiosyncratic behaviors that may or may not be viewed as communicative by clinicians who do not know the child, and direct feedback as to kinds of activities and interactions that seem to be most successful in eliciting communicative behavior. (See Schuler, Peck, Willard, & Theimer, 1989; Watson, Lord, Schaeffer, & Schopler, 1989.) Furthermore, assessment should take into account caregivers' perceptions of their child's communicative needs relative to independent functioning and social-emotional growth, and family needs, relative to a child's communicative competence.

For very young children, communication assessment clearly is not a one time occurrence. Children with autism may show situation-specific communicative skills, relative to the types of routines and interactions that they are engaged in (Prizant & Schuler, 1987a). Furthermore, some children demonstrate an uneven rate or "spurts" in development in the preschool years. Thus, communication assessment must be an ongoing process to carefully monitor the growth of communicative competence and to take into account the range of abilities that may be demonstrated in different contexts and with different persons (Prizant & Bailey, 1992).

Content of Assessment

Because autism is a developmental disorder, information on normal language and communication development offers an organizational framework for the assessment and enhancement of language and communication (Wetherby & Prizant, 1992). In a more detailed discussion of the application of developmental information, we delineated three general principles that the developmental literature has contributed to communication assessment and enhancement (Prizant & Wetherby, 1989). First, communication development involves continuity from pre-verbal to verbal communication. That is, the development of preverbal communication is a necessary precursor to the development of the intentional use of language to communicate. Second, development of competence in communication is the outcome of a developmental inter-action of cognitive, social-affective, and linguistic abilities. A child's profile across these domains should provide the basis for clinical deci-sion-making. Third, in a developmental model, all behavior should be viewed in reference to the child's relative level of functioning across developmental domains. Many of the behavior problems displayed by autistic children can be understood as expressions of communicative intent if they are interpreted with a child's communication limitations and developmental level in mind (Prizant & Wetherby, 1987).

Based on these principles, a developmental approach to assessment and intervention of communication obligates clinicians or educators to have a practical understanding of normal development, to ascertain a child's developmental level across cognitive, social, and linguistic do-mains, and to target in intervention the communicative and conceptual basis of conventional preverbal, and, if possible, linguistic communica-tion. In a review of 43 language intervention studies with autistic and severely handicapped individuals, Bryen and Joyce (1985) found that only 7 studies considered social factors and only 5 studies considered children's level of symbolic functioning in planning intervention ap-proaches. Assessment procedures used in the vast majority of the stud-ies consisted primarily of collecting baseline data on the presence or absence of specific language forms (e.g., number of speech sounds, number of words, specific grammatical forms). It is our hope that intervention studies of the next decade will consider developmental issues in baseline assessment in order to better evaluate the effective-ness and efficiency of intervention.

Application of a Developmental Framework

In the first few years of life, a child's behavior becomes increas-ingly more deliberate and goal-directed, showing increased evidence of organization, planning, and foresight. This leads to the ability to plan behavior through symbolic thought, evident in a child's language and play. Because children with autism experience cognitive, social, and affective impairments, the normal emergence of language and play abilities is disrupted. However, information on communication and language development of children without disabilities can provide a framework for assessing communication abilities and prioritizing intervention goals. Table 5-1 presents an overview of the major stages in communication and language development, with approximate developmental age ranges for each stage. This discussion will focus on the expression of communication and language. The reader is referred to Lord (1985) for a discussion of language comprehension, Dawson and Galpert (1986) for a discussion of social behavior, and Westby (1988) for a discussion of symbolic functioning.

Preverbal Communication

Before using words, normally developing children learn to communicate intentionally with preverbal gestures and sounds, to reference objects and events with indicative gestures (e.g., pointing), and to use conventional signals that have shared meanings (Bates, O'Connell, & Shore, 1987). These preverbal communicative achievements provide the foundation for the emergence of language. Dore (1986) suggested that the caregiver "induces" intent in the infant within preverbal dialogues in which affective states are shared. These early social interactions involving shared affective experiences lead to the infant's awareness of the effect that his/her behavior can have on others (Bruner, 1981; Dore, 1986).

At about 9 to 10 months of age, children begin to use gestures and/or sounds to communicate intentionally. That is, particular signals are used deliberately to have a preplanned effect on another person (Bates, 1979). Bruner (1981) suggested that there are three "innate communicative intentions" that emerge during the first year of life:

1. *Behavioral regulation,* which includes signals used to regulate another's behavior for purposes of obtaining or restricting environmental goals;
2. *Social interaction,* which includes signals used to attract and maintain another's attention to oneself for affiliative purposes; and
3. *Joint attention,* which includes acts used to direct another's attention for purposes of sharing the focus on an entity or event.

Table 5-1. Major Developmental Stages in Language Acquisition*

Intentional Communication: 9–13 months
- Uses gestures and/or sounds to communicate with clear evidence of intentionality
- Communicates to regulate other's behaviors, to engage in social interaction, and to reference joint attention

First Words: 13–18 months
- Increases use of gestures and sound in coordination to communicate intent
- Repairs unsuccessful communicative interactions by repeating, modifying the form, or using an alternative strategy
- Uses a small number of conventional signals referentially, i.e., to refer to objects or classes of objects
- Shows slow vocabulary growth with some attrition of vocabulary; inventory of words usually does not exceed 10 to 20 single words at one time
- Most words are used to encode the semantic relations of existence, nonexistence, recurrence, and rejection

First Word Combinations: 18–30 months
- Shows a sudden surge in vocabulary growth from a few dozen to several hundred words; vocabulary attrition should no longer be evident
- Uses imitation as a predominant strategy in language learning
- Engages in conversation, i.e., discourse functions emerge as child produces more utterances that are contingent upon the previous speaker's turn
- Provides and requests information about objects or events remote in time or place from the immediate context
- Uses words and word combinations for predication, i.e., to encode a state or quality attributed to one entity or a relationship attributed to two or more entities
- Shows expansion of single-word semantic relations (e.g., action, attribute, denial, location, possession)
- Uses word combinations to encode semantic relations (e.g., action + object, agent + action, attribute + entity, action + location, possessor + possession, etc.)

Sentence Grammar: 30 months–5 years
- Uses grammatical morphemes (e.g., prepositions, tense markers, plural endings, pronouns, articles)
- Uses modalities of simple sentences (i.e., uses word order for declarative, negative, imperative, and interrogative constructions)
- Develops semantic relational terms to encode spatial, dimensional, temporal, causal, quantity, color, age, and other relations
- Develops increasing sentence complexity (i.e., elaboration of phrase and clause structure used in simple and complex sentence constructions)

Discourse Grammar: 5–8 years
- Uses grammar and vocabulary to express text cohesion (i.e., to make a group of sentences hang together by setting up transitions between sentences and clarifying shifts in reference from one clause or sentence to another)
- Develops metalinguistic awareness of language structure and meaning (i.e., ability to focus attention to both language form and content; develops skills such as making grammatical judgments, resolving lexical ambiguity, using multiple meanings of words in humor, and segmenting words into phonemes)

*From Bates, O'Connell, & Shore, 1987; Owens, 1992; Van Kleeck, 1984; Wetherby, Cain, Yonclas, & Walker, 1988; Wetherby & Prizant, 1989.

In a study of intentional communication of 15 normally developing children from the prelinguistic to the multiword stage, Wetherby, Cain, Yonclas, and Walker (1988) found that all the children used intentional communicative signals for behavioral regulation, social interaction, and joint attention functions during the prelinguistic stage. Thus, before the emergence of words, normally developing children are able to use signals intentionally to communicate these three major functions.

The sophistication of communicative behaviors used to express these functions increases along a number of dimensions from the prelinguistic to the multiword stage. The gestures that children first use at about 9 months are contact gestures, that is, the child's hand comes in physical contact with an object or another person. Examples of contact gestures are giving an object, showing an object, and pushing an adult's hand. Examples of distal gestures, which emerge at about 11 months, are open-hand reaching, distant pointing, and waving (Bates *et al.,* 1987). Bates (1979) has found that giving and showing are necessary precursors to the use of pointing to reference joint attention, and that these gestures are highly correlated with the subsequent emergence of naming. In other words, children first learn to reference with gestures and then with words.

Verbal Communication

There is a gradual transition from preverbal sounds and gestures to first words. Between 9 and 13 months children begin to use conventional sounds to signify a specific communicative function, such as "mama" as a general purpose request for objects, and to make a predictable point in an episode, such as "bye bye" when closing a book and "uh-oh" when knocking down blocks. At this stage children are able to repair communication breakdowns by repeating their message or using different sounds or gestures to get their point across. At about 13 months children begin using a small number of words that are symbolic or referential, that is, labels which are used to refer to an object or class of objects. New word acquisition is very slow at this stage, and highly variable across children, and it is not unusual for old words to drop out of a child's vocabulary as a new word comes in, which sometimes causes concern to parents. Between 12 and 18 months children show an increase in the rate of communicating, in the use of sounds in combination with gestures, and in the use of consonants in multisyllabic utterances (Wetherby *et al.*, 1988).

At about 18 months there is a sudden surge in vocabulary growth from acquisition of about one new word a week, to several new words a day, and major changes can be seen in language abilities from 18 to 24 months. At this stage children begin to produce word combinations and to predicate, that is, to describe states and qualities of objects. Semantic meanings expressed in single words and word combinations have been found to be similar across languages and to include agents, actions, attributes, location, possession, disappearance, and denial (Bates *et al.*, 1987). At this stage, children begin requesting information, bringing up topics about things that are remote in place and time, and maintaining a topic for several turns, and thus are truly engaging in conversation.

Between 20 and 30 months children acquire the basics of sentence grammar, including morphology, the organization of words; and syntax, the organization of sentences (Owens, 1992). Children begin to construct more adult-like sentence forms for declaratives, negatives, imperatives, and interrogatives. With continued rapid vocabulary growth, children acquire semantic relational terms to encode concepts such as position, size, colors, numerosity, time, and causality. These advances in grammar and semantics contribute to the child's advancing conversational competence.

Between 3 and 5 years of age children's grammar is primarily organized at a sentence level and further development is seen in sentence complexity. Children learn to combine two or more simple sentences into one complex sentence by conjoining (i.e., combining two main clauses with a conjunction) and embedding (i.e., modifying an element of a main clause by inserting a subordinate clause). By about age 5 children begin to develop discourse grammar. This involves the ability to construct a text—a group of sentences that unfold a plot, by setting up transitions between sentences and clarifying shifts in reference from one sentence to another. Emerging discourse grammar is apparent in a child's developing ability to tell stories about personal events, to retell stories that have been told to them, or to make up new stories. In addition to language achievements, children begin to develop metalinguistic skills, which involve the ability to focus awareness on the units and rules of language and reflect upon language as a system for communication. A child should enter school with a rich foundation of spoken language skills to succeed in academics (Van Kleeck, 1984).

Assigning a Communication/Language Stage

The developmental framework presented in Table 5-1 can be used to identify a child's language level, which, in turn, contributes to selection and prioritization of intervention goals. However, determining the true language and communication level of a child with autism may be difficult, particularly for a child who has the memory capacity to learn language forms with only limited understanding of the use or meanings of these forms. It is not simply a matter of determining that a child is preverbal or verbal, but rather, examining how the child uses gestures, sounds, words (spoken or signed) and word combinations. A child's expressive language should be compared with his/her symbolic level in other domains to obtain an accurate picture of symbolic functioning.

Four major questions should be considered in assigning a language level. First, what gestures, sounds, and/or words does a child use that serve a communicative purpose and are these used intentionally (Wetherby & Prizant, 1989)? Second, does a child use words, and if so, do the words have referential meaning? That is, does the child use words accurately to refer to specific objects and not use that word inappropriately to refer to other things? Children who use words or word combinations communicatively, but not referentially, will typically cycle through their repertoire of utterances in an attempt to request an object until they happen upon the name and attain the goal. For example, a child with autism was able to request objects and actions with gestures and signs and had an inventory of about 10 different signs, mainly labels for food items. In trying to request a cracker that was out of his reach, he first signed "want nut." Without success, he persisted by signing "want apple," then "want cookie," and finally "want cracker." This child was able to use these signs for a communicative function (i.e., behavior regulation), but was not using them referentially, therefore, his message was unclear. His language level is best characterized as early emerging first words, rather than first word combinations.

Third, how many different words and word combinations does the child use referentially? For a child who is producing spontaneous and/

or echolalic utterances, the inventory of utterances (i.e., number of different utterances) used referentially may be a more accurate measure of language level than utterance length or complexity. If a child uses less than 10 to 20 different spontaneous utterances, it is likely that the child's overall language level is within first words, rather than first word combinations, because his/her repertoire may consist primarily of routinized forms. And fourth, for a child who is using word combinations, does the child use the individual words alone and in combination with other words, or is an utterance equivalent to a single word? For example, a child with autism used over 50 different nouns referentially, some in the phrase "wanna have some _____ please," to request items. These phrases were equivalent to two-word combinations for this child. This child also used a number of delayed echolalic utterances, such as "stop doing that" to protest and "time to say goodbye" to greet, which were equivalent to single words because they were used only as single units. This child's language level is best characterized as emerging first word combinations.

Language skills that are at or listed below a child's overall language level (See Table 5-1) would take priority in intervention. For the child described above at the first words stage, a developmental approach would place priority on expanding the range of communicative functions, developing the use of a small number of words (signs) referentially, and developing a variety of semantic relations (e.g., existence, nonexistence, recurrence, rejection) which can later be used in word combinations. For the second child described above at the first word combination stage, emphasis should be placed on developing the skills listed below this stage and then in this stage (e.g., if the child uses all three communicative functions, proceed to discourse functions). Because this child's language level appears much higher on the surface, it is tempting to target more complex grammatical structures to increase utterance length (e.g., pronouns; see Fay, 1979). However, this child does not yet have the pragmatic and semantic language base for the sentence grammar stage.

Recently, we have completed national standardization of an assessment instrument, the *Communication and Symbolic Behavior Scales* (Wetherby & Prizant, 1993), which addresses many of the issues regarding content and context of assessment discussed above. The CSBS provides a profile of strengths and needs across communication, symbolic, and social–affective abilities for children up to five years of age. This profile provides direct implications for intervention (Wetherby & Prizant, 1992).

Regardless of the procedures used, establishing a child's true level of communication and related abilities leads directly to intervention goals. In addition to increasing complexity and range of communicative skills, those skills which lead directly to precluding or ameliorating behavior problems should be a priority and thus be targeted in appropriate contexts.

COMMUNICATION ENHANCEMENT

Contexts of Communication Enhancement

Appropriateness of services to preschool children with autism is determined by content of programming and by the contexts of educational and clinical services.[†] Contexts of treatment and educational services are determined by a number of factors including: the chronological age of the child, mobility of caregivers, availability of services to preschool children at a center or a school, and, when services are available, the ability of professionals to work in home environments as well as in centers or educational environments. Treatment approaches fall under two general headings: home- and center-based approaches. Of course, aspects of both home- and center-based approaches may be included in a coordinated system of services.

Home-based approaches may be directed to the child and/or to the caregiver in enhancing children's communication abilities. Home-based approaches may be the primary strategy for very young children (e.g., younger than three years of age), or may be an adjunct to services provided in a center or educational setting. For caregivers of very young children who live a distance from treatment or educational settings, or who have limited ability to bring children to a center, a home-based approach may be more convenient for the family. Furthermore, the provision of services within the home allows the early interventionist or educator to observe, and take advantage of regular family routines as a vehicle for communication enhancement. Professionals may suggest modifications of the physical environment in order to help create natural opportunities and needs for communication. Other family members including siblings and grandparents can become involved in a setting that is familiar and comfortable to them. The major advantage of home-based approaches is their ecological soundness; that is, the services that are being provided directly to the family and the child are more likely to meet their needs, and acquired communicative abilities are more likely to be used in daily routines. This is especially crucial for children with autism, whose situation-specific learning style often results in generalization problems. Professionals also are able to get a more accurate picture of the child's abilities, and the challenges parents face. In most states, preschool programs, whether they be specifically for children with autism, or integrated noncategorical programs, are available for children 3 to 5 years of age. Some programs include periodic home visits as part of the services provided. However, for children younger than age 3, home-based approaches may be the primary vehicle for service delivery.

Center-based approaches also may be directed to the child, parent or both. Centers may include programs in schools, hospitals, or community-based clinics. In some states, preschool programs for children 3 to 5 years of age may provide half-day or full-day services in educational settings. However, center-based approaches also are relevant for children under three years of age and for this population may provide particular benefits for both the family and the child. Attendance at a center-based program may help some caregivers to combat their feeling of isolation. Many centers run parent and sibling groups which provide an emotionally supportive forum to express concerns and to share experiences. In specific reference to understanding communication problems and enhancing their children's communication abilities, caregivers can compare notes and share "home made" strategies. They also may learn to understand their role as an advocate for their child, an important skill considering the coming years of potential frustration in finding appropriate services.

Center-based approaches also provide opportunities for a child to have varied experiences with other children and adults in the center or in community sites. Community-based activities provide contexts for enhancing functional communication skills in natural settings. Programs also can provide contact with other children in regularly scheduled activities or routines, providing opportunities for targeting specific language and social-communicative goals. When such programs are available, parents may be afforded much needed time to attend to other obligations or to get a "breather" from the demands of caring for their child. Some centers also offer respite services enabling families to live a more normal life. For more demanding children, these interactive support services often result in the family being able to maintain a child in the home setting rather than resorting to residential placement. Furthermore, family members may have more energy for interacting with the affected child when it is not a full-time occurrence.

The effectiveness of home- or center-based approaches for communication enhancement depends largely on the degree of active involvement and cooperation on the part of the family (Rossetti, 1986). Approaches focusing solely on the child often do not address life-span issues for the family, or immediate stresses experienced by the family. Approaches that empower families by including them as partners in the early intervention and educational process have a much greater chance of having an immediate and lasting impact (National Center for Clinical Infant Programs, 1985). Thus, caregivers must become actively involved. The degree of active involvement may vary, however, depending upon family composition and resources (Powell, Hecimovic, & Christensen, 1992).

Caregiver Involvement in Communication Enhancement

In considering approaches to intervention, a family systems approach is advocated (Bristol, 1985) in designing appropriate intervention strategies for enhancing language and communication ability. Within this framework, parents are viewed as partners in the process rather than as patients that need to be treated or dictated to (Bristol, 1985). Furthermore, this approach recognizes the impact that a severe disability such as autism can have on the day-to-day functioning of the family (Powell *et al.*, 1992; Prizant & Meyer, in press). Thus, intervention planning must include family member as active participants as well as addressing the needs of both the affected child and the family. In explaining this approach, Bristol (1985) noted that "intervention that affects only the child or even the child and one parent is not considered appropriate. The entire family is seen as one of an interactive, interdependent set of systems "nested" within each other. The child affects and is affected by the entire family system . . . " (p. 49). Thus, success of a language and communication enhancement program for preschool children with autism cannot be measured solely in terms of the child's progress. Family involvement and family adaptation to the child also must be taken into account. A carefully coordinated multidisciplinary approach to communication enhancement and early intervention is crucial to the goal of meeting a broad range of needs for the child and family (Powers, 1992).

Family systems principles are especially relevant for efforts to enhance language and communication, for it is limitations in communication and social interaction skills that create the most significant barriers between the child and other family members. Conversely, progress in language and communication development may have a positive impact on a child's social, emotional, and adaptive functioning and foster more successful and mutually satisfying interactions between the child and other family members (Prizant & Meyer, in press).

It is our belief that caregivers, when given the appropriate resources and support, can be the most effective agents in enhancing their children's language and communicative development. Thus, professionals must play a somewhat different role in working with families of preschool children than families of older children being served in full day programs within educational settings. Professionals need to work closely with caregivers toward accomplishing a variety of goals. These include:

1. Developing an accurate picture of a child's communication ability and profile of related abilities.
2. Developing strategies for simplifying and modifying linguistic and social-communicative behavior with a child to ensure more successful interactions (see Prizant & Schuler, 1987b for further discussion).
3. Identifying regularly occurring routines both within the home as well as in the center or educational environment that provides contexts and motivating activities that may facilitate communication development.
4. Identifying the types and amount of information, and/or training needed by caregivers to enhance communication.

In approaching the first goal, assessment information should be discussed with caregivers relative to a child's strengths and weaknesses. Typical relative strengths for preschoolers with autism may include a child's proficiency to engage in activities with visual-spatial materials, to develop recognition of routine play interactions and anticipate steps of an activity, to engage in motor activities, and so forth. Weaknesses may include limited ability to attend to and/or comprehend language, to use conventional signals to communicate, and to persist if communication is not successful or to communicate for social purposes (i.e., functions of social interaction or joint attention).

Professionals may use a variety of strategies in helping parents to fulfill their role as primary enhancers of communication. Strategies used depend upon ability of the caregiver to be involved in different activities, or to modify family and caregiving routines. Different activities may vary in time commitment, the degree to which interactions in the home need to be modified, and flexibility of the family schedule and lifestyle. Strategies in working with caregivers also vary as to how directive or non-directive they are in their communicative style. Behavioral approaches in working with parents around communication issues traditionally have been more directive, where parents are taught to identify specific behaviors, and to apply various behavioral procedures to increase or decrease the behavior in question (Schreibman, Koegel, Mills, & Burke, 1984). Less directive approaches are geared toward helping caregivers discover the types of interactions and modifications in their own behavior that are most successful for maintaining and enhancing communicative interactions. The choice of directive vs. non-directive approaches will be determined, to some extent, by the challenges presented by a child's behavior, as well as by parental style. Thus, professionals should be knowledgeable about the range of approaches available (see Marfo, 1990, for further discussion). Parents with children with more challenging and difficult-to-manage behaviors and/or limited attentional abilities may respond initially to more directive approaches whereas those with children with less challenging behaviors and greater attention and motivation to communicate may respond more positively to non-directive approaches. Similarly, some caregivers may feel more comfortable with one type of approach versus others.

Caregivers with greater amounts of time and flexibility also may benefit from educational approaches, in which they become involved with other parents in learning general principles for communication enhancement, and applying such principles with their children. One example of this is the *Hanen Early Language Parent Program* (Manolson, 1992), which has been modified for parents of children with autism (Weitzman & Mayerovitch, 1987). In this relatively non-directive approach, parents are taught basic principles of communication enhancement including developing an accurate picture of their children's communication abilities, learning how to recognize and follow up on children's initiations, to expand turntaking, and to use a variety of educational and creative media for motivating and enhancing communication. The Hanen Program does not focus primary attention on individual children, nor on highly prescriptive techniques, and thus requires caregivers to take the major responsibility in developing an understanding of their children's communication development, and to develop strategies and seize opportunities for enhancing communication in natural interactions.

Consideration of the Nature of Communication Problems in Autism

Understanding the nature of the communication problems characteristic of autism contributes greatly to the design of education programs (Prizant & Schuler, 1987b; Prizant & Wetherby, 1989; Quill, in press). Because current definitions of autism emphasize the social-affective and communication impairments as primary (Denckla, 1986; Fein *et al.*, 1986), language and communication intervention should address competence in these domains, rather than merely teach isolated verbal or nonverbal behaviors. The major communication goals that should be emphasized based on the nature of the communication problems in autism are outlined in Table 5-2. The goals in Table 5-2 are not inconsistent with the developmental framework presented in Table 5-1, but rather offer some special considerations for the child with autism.

Several studies have demonstrated that children with autism in the early stages of communication and language development do initiate communication but show a restricted range of communicative functions (Curcio, 1978; Mundy, Sigman, Ungerer, & Sherman, 1986; Wetherby & Prutting, 1984; Wetherby, Yonclas, & Bryan, 1989). These studies have found that autistic children communicate primarily or exclusively

. Priority Goals for Communication Intervention with Autistic Children*

Expand Repertoire of Communicative Functions

.egulate another's behavior
- to request action, request object, protest

2. Engage in social interaction
- to request social routine, greet, call, request permission, show off

3. Reference joint attention
- to label or comment on objects or actions, request information, and provide or request clarification

Develop Sophistication of Communicative Means for Each Function

1. Develop persistence and use of repair strategies
2. Replace aberrant communicative behavior with socially acceptable means
3. Improve readability of communicative means
4. Develop symbolic level of communicative means
   - from contact to distal gestures
   - from depictive to symbolic gestures (including signs)
   - from presymbolic sounds to referential words
5. Develop ability to segment echolalic utterances into meaningful units and produce creative word combinations

Enhance Reciprocity of Communication

1. Develop ability to participate in turn-taking interactions
2. Develop ability to consider what information is needed by the listener to understand the message and to revise message as needed to clarify intentions or referent for listener
3. Develop ability to collaborate on topics in conversation based on conventional meanings

*Adapted from Prizant & Wetherby, *Topics in Language Disorders, 9,* No. 1, p. 9, with permission of Aspen Publishers, Inc., December, 1988.

for behavioral regulation functions and show limited ability to communicate for social interaction or joint attention functions. While normally developing children use all of these functions before using words, some children with autism may use words but communicate only for behavior regulation (i.e., requesting objects/actions, protesting).

Wetherby (1986) suggested that the first emerging category of intentional communication for autistic children is regulating others' behavior, while referencing joint attention emerges later, presumably because of the differing social underpinnings of these abilities. Based on this progression, the first goal in intervention should be to teach a child to communicate in order to regulate another's behavior—to request actions, request objects, and protest, if the child does not communicate these functions. For very young or more severely impaired children, the first step is to establish motivations to communicate (objects and activities that the child does and does not like), and then have the child communicate to the adult as a means to obtain or reject objects or others' actions. Child-initiated communication may be encouraged by structuring the environment and interactions; for example, by placing desired objects so that they are out of the child's reach or in containers the child cannot open, engaging the child in an activity where adult assistance is needed, and offering the child objects that the child likes and does not like (Prizant & Wetherby, 1988). The consistent use of predictable activity routines, involving both nonsocial goals (e.g., requesting objects) and more social goals (e.g., requesting assistance) is important for establishing and motivating spontaneous communication (Prizant, 1982). As the child progresses, adults can introduce a variety of social routines or games that involve adult–child turn-taking interactions with exchangeable roles, such as "peek-a-boo" and "I'm gonna get you" (see Snyder-McLean, Solomonson, McLean, & Sack, 1984). These games or routines can use a paradigm similar to requesting action for assistance, and facilitate the use of communication for the social end of attracting attention to oneself. After a child begins communicating to engage in social interaction, the adult can devise turn-taking interactions that introduce or manipulate objects systematically to facilitate the child's use of communication to direct attention to an object or event.

We recommend that all early language and communication goals address one of the three major communicative functions—behavior regulation, social interaction, or joint attention. Natural reinforcers that are consistent with the child's intention should be used. Consider whether the child's act serves to regulate another's behavior, to engage in social interaction, or to reference joint attention, and then respond naturally to that function (Wetherby, 1986). If the child is requesting or protesting (i.e., rejecting) an object, the natural reinforcer is to offer or remove the object. If the child is greeting or calling, the natural reinforcer is to attend to the child. If the child is labeling or commenting, the natural reinforcer is to attend to the object or event. For a more thorough discussion of communicative functions, refer to Wetherby and Prizant (1989).

Communicative means are the behaviors used to express communicative intentions and may include gestures, sounds, or words. Parameters to be considered in developing the sophistication of communicative means for children with autism are listed in Table 5-2. Children with autism may not persist in communicating if initial communicative efforts are unsuccessful. Therefore, a primary consideration in intervention should be to develop the use of flexible strategies to repair unsuccessful communicative attempts by repeating, modifying, or using alternative means.

Some children may use socially unacceptable behavior, such as aggression or self-injury, as an attempt to communicate. The primary goal when dealing with a socially unacceptable expression of intent is to replace such challenging behavior with more socially acceptable forms for expressing that communicative function (e.g., a more acceptable way to protest or call attention to oneself), rather than simply attempting to eradicate or extinguish such behavior (Donnellan *et al.*, 1984; Schuler & Prizant, 1987). Short-term considerations include the child's immediate safety and the safety of others. Long-term considerations involve the acceptability of a child's behavior in social contexts. Research has demonstrated that these problem behaviors may be reduced significantly when children and even adults learn to use more acceptable means to serve the same function e.g., protest, requesting assistance, etc; (Carr & Durand, 1986; Smith, 1985). Older individuals with autism with limited repertoires of conventional communicative behaviors may display volatile maladaptive behaviors when they cannot successfully communicate, for example, to express that they are frustrated or bored with an activity, or to indicate distress over a routine being disrupted. To prevent this developmental outcome, communicative goals should be emphasized in young autistic children to provide for a variety of appropriate alternative means to express their intentions.

Another important consideration is the readability of the child's communicative behavior, that is, how clear the child's intent is to the communicative partner. The familiarity of the communicative partner will affect readability. Children with autism often use idiosyncratic means of communicating; therefore, intervention goals need to address conventionality of means. Echolalia and metaphorical language may be used with clear intent but have limited effectiveness if their origin or referent is not shared by the listener (Prizant & Rydell, 1993). Readability is also dependent on the explicitness of the signals used in expressing meanings and intents. More generalized conventional preverbal communication (e.g., pointing, head shakes, head nods) is typically limited in very young children, requiring that communicative partners use contextual and other nonlinguistic cues in inferring intent.

Impairments in symbolic skills are also primary to autism (APA, 1987) and affect the child's development of play as well as communication. The symbolic level (or level of sophistication) of communicative means should be targeted in intervention along with the development of play skills. However, we recommend that symbolic level of communicative means not take priority over persistence, social acceptability, and readability of means. In regard to preverbal gestures, dimensions of development to be considered include contact to distal gestures and depictive to symbolic gestures. Preverbal sounds used with communicative intent should be developed before teaching speech. Movement to symbolic communicative means should be made in the child's strongest modality, that is to referential words, spoken or signed.

For children with autism, sophistication of means is not simply a matter of using words or using longer sentences. It is also a matter of generating creative utterances. This is of particular concern because most children with autism do develop speech progress through stages of using echolalia (Prizant, 1983). Echolalia has been found to represent a continuum of behaviors, ranging from noncommunicative to clearly intentional serving a variety of communicative functions (Schuler & Prizant, 1985). Intervention efforts should exploit the child's communicative use of echolalia by responding to the child's intentions. Strategies to help the child segment echolalic utterances into smaller meaningful units should be used (see Prizant, 1987; 1988). Thus, even simple two- to three-word utterances that are creative word combinations should be considered more sophisticated in linguistic form than longer memorized language "chunks" (see Prizant & Rydell, 1993, for a detailed consideration of echolalia and forms of unconventional verbal behavior).

In contrast to language development of normally developing children, children with autism may show discrepancies in the sophistication of communicative means to express the three major communicative functions (Prizant & Wetherby, 1988; Wetherby, 1986). The developmental interaction of communicative functions and means should be considered (Prizant & Schuler, 1987a; Prizant & Wetherby, 1988; Wetherby, 1986). New communicative functions should be taught initially through simple means within the child's repertoire. More conventional, socially acceptable, and sophisticated means should be mapped onto established communicative functions. For a particular child, an appropriate goal for one function might be the use of single- or multi-word utterances while an appropriate goal for another function might be the use of a contact gesture to replace disruptive behavior.

Children with autism also show difficulties with the reciprocity of communication, ranging from impairments in synchronizing and regulating turn-taking to making poor judgments about what the listener needs to know to interpret their message (Dawson & Galpert, 1986). Children with greater abilities who reach a discourse level of communication show difficulties with conversational contingency. They may initiate topics without identifying the referent and have difficulties revising a message to clarify what the listener needs to know. Maintaining a topic of joint focus may be problematic when conversing with children with autism. For example, they may engage in a particular dialogue to complete a ritual rather than to share information. They may group words or follow topics by the way words sound rather than by their meaning, making it hard for the listener to identify or maintain the topic. The dimensions of reciprocity that need to be considered are listed in Table 5-2. (See Klinger & Dawson, 1992, for strategies to increase reciprocity and joint attention.)

One important principle derived from the developmental literature is that successful communicative interactions involve the cooperative effort of two or more people (Prizant & Wetherby, 1988). Therefore, intervention goals should address the level of the dyad, or small group, rather than the individual child. Changes in the behavior of both members of the dyad are necessary to enhance communication development (MacDonald, 1985; 1989). Rather than viewing communication intervention as "fixing" the child with autism, intervention should be conceptualized as enhancing communicative interactions between the child and various partners including family members and peers who are significant to the child. For very young children, the emphasis should be on adult–child interactions involving caregivers. When beginning child–child interactions, linguistic and communicative demands should be minimized to ensure successful social interactions. The progression of communicative functions suggested by Wetherby (1986) may be replicated with peers following success with adults, beginning with behavior regulation functions (e.g., requesting an action or object from a peer). The use of simple communicative means to express functions that the child is able to use with adults should be targeted with peers.

Consideration of Broader Contexts of Communication

Children younger than three years of age typically have their daily life experiences within the family or extended family context. As noted, many children from 3 to 5 years of age typically will experience more varied contexts and a broader social network as they receive regularly scheduled services in centers or educational settings. As a child's life contexts expand, so do communicative needs as well as opportunities for communication enhancement. Professionals must work closely with parents in recognizing a child's increasing communication needs as his or her living environments expand. Performing ecological inventories (Falvey, 1986) may be helpful in targeting communication goals as discrepancies are observed between a child's current communication abilities, and abilities needed to be most independent in various contexts. Such increased competences may include the ability to interact with and communicate to peers, the ability to communicate to a wider variety of adults in a conventional and socially acceptable manner, and the ability to develop some internalized sense of daily routine. Many programs for preschool children with autism are now using integration strategies with normally developing peers as a primary component of educational placement. The efficacy of integration strategies has been supported by a variety of studies with young children with autism (Goldstein & Strain, 1988). Integration strategies may include direct training of peers to initiate and maintain interactions with young children with autism. Clearly, the potential benefit of nondisabled peer models for communication and social enhancement must be explored in current and future programming for preschool children. It is likely that by being exposed to good social and communicative role models, children with autism will progress from idiosyncratic and unconventional communicative means, to more conventional and effective means.

Additional Considerations

Educators and clinicians face additional challenges in planning for communication enhancement. These include the use of nonspeech communication systems, and how communication enhancement programs are to be organized and structured.

?ech Communication

ιportant decisions regarding communication enhancement include whether a child can benefit from the introduction of an augmentative or nonspeech communication system, and the timing of introducing a child to a formal communication system. The following questions should be considered when making decisions about implementing formal communication systems.

1. Is a child communicating intentionally with natural gestures (conventional or unconventional)?
2. Does a child demonstrate frustration frequently, resulting in behavior problems or withdrawal due to communicative limitations?
3. Is a child's current expressive communicative repertoire unconventional or idiosyncratic?
4. Is a child communicating as effectively as he may be capable of without the possible implementation of a nonspeech communication system?
5. Does a child demonstrate limited motor control or proficiency for speech production, yet demonstrate clear communicative intent?
6. Does a child demonstrate some preference for attending to pictures, or demonstrate the capability of comprehending pictures?

If any answer to questions 1 through 5 is affirmative, serious consideration should be given to nonspeech communication. If the answer to question 6 is affirmative, a pictorial system may be the system of preference (Mirenda, 1985).

Deciding to implement nonspeech communication systems in communication enhancement, whether they be gestural systems such as natural gestures or sign language, or pictorial systems such as communication boards or books, is not a black or white decision. Our current knowledge suggests it should not be so (Mirenda & Schuler, 1988). That is, children may be introduced gradually to pictures as communication aids, or to gestures or signs within the context of specific activities on a trial basis. Intensive practice may occur in specific activities during the day, with careful monitoring as to the child's acquisition of specific communicative means in those activities. Contraindicators for nonspeech communication systems may be a child's inability to attend to two-dimensional representations, or lack of intentional, even primitive means of communication; for picture systems and problems in motor planning and motor control for sign systems. Because many children develop behavioral problems related to their frustration in communication, or as a means to express intent, nonspeech communication systems should always be a consideration for any child with autism 2½ to 3 who is not developing speech. Even for children who are in early stages of language acquisition, or who are echolalic, augmenting communication with pictorial or sign systems may facilitate development of speech and language. However, if the introduction of a nonspeech system causes sufficient confusion or anxiety for a child, even after a trial period, another system should be attempted, or efforts postponed. Furthermore, unless the decision to implement nonspeech systems is supported by caregivers, and carried through to other environments, it may not be justified, and may even cause friction between caregivers and professionals. Professionals must work carefully with parents to help them understand that introducing nonspeech systems does not mean that speech is "being given up on," and that research indicates that nonspeech systems may actually facilitate speech acquisition (Mirenda & Schuler, 1988).

Structuring Communication Enhancement Programs for Preschoolers

The value of consistency, predictability and an understandable routine structure cannot be overestimated for children with autism. This is true even at the preschool level where efforts can begin to help children develop some "cognitive comfort" based upon the ability to plan and anticipate relative to daily schedules. For home-based programs, professionals can help parents provide "guideposts" or obvious cues to help their children develop a sense of the routine of the day. This may be done initially around common family routines such as mealtime, bathing, grooming and bedtime. For older preschoolers, additional structure can be provided through half-day or full-day programs at a center or school.

Strategies to help children understand, anticipate, and even request past or future activities should include the use of simple redundant language, gestures, other auditory cues (songs, bells, etc.), and, when appropriate, objects or visual aids such as pictures on schedules or timeboards. The use of these types of strategies takes advantage of learning strengths, and goes a long way in reducing confusion and frustration that often result in behavioral difficulties for young children. Quill (in press) provides detailed information regarding the use of learning strengths in educational programming.

Additionally, clinicians and educators should recognize that preschool children with autism have the same needs as any preschool children. Learning environments should foster a sense of competence, and trust in others, which provides the foundation for further learning and development of communication and social-affective skills. Rigid training approaches that focus on behavioral control and compliance training, without encouraging initiated spontaneous communication and playful exploration may be counterproductive to later development. Lethargy and passivity often observed in adolescents and adults with autism presumably could be precluded, to some extent, if young children are given a sense of active involvement and communicative control using the strategies we have discussed.

CONCLUSION

The preschool years are a time of great potential growth for young children with autism, but remain a time of great stress for families and great challenge to professionals. We believe that preschool approaches, regardless of environments in which they are undertaken, should emphasize communication and social-affective competence. Abilities in these areas provide the foundation for learning with and from others, and developing positive affective relationships and a sense of self as a competent social participant. With a continued focus on these areas in preschool services, both families and professionals can expect more positive outcomes for preschool children with autism and their caregivers.

REFERENCES

American Psychiatric Association (1987). *Diagnostic and Statistical Manual of Mental Disorders* (3rd ed., rev.) Washington, DC: Author.

Bates, E. (1979). *The emergence of symbols: Cognition and communication in infancy.* New York: Academic Press.

Bates, E., O'Connell, B., & Shore, C. (1987). Language and communication in infancy. In J. Osofsky (Ed.), *Handbook of infant development.* New York: Wiley.

Bristol, M. (1985). Designing programs for young developmentally disabled children: A family systems approach to autism. *Remedial and Special Education, 6*(4) 46–53.

Brown, L., Branston, M. B., Hamre-Nietupski, S., Pumpian, I., Certo, N., & Gruenewald, L. (1979). A strategy for developing chronological age-appropriate and functional curricular content for severely handicapped adolescents and young adults. *Journal of Special Education, 13,* 81–90.

Bruner, J. (1981). The social context of language acquisition. *Language and Communication, 1,* 155–178.

Bruner, J. (1983). *In search of mind: Essays in autobiography.* New York: Basic Books.

Bryen, D., & Joyce, D. (1985). Language intervention with the severely handicapped: A decade of research. *Journal of Special Education, 19,* 7–39.

Carr, E., & Durand, V. (1986). Reducing behavior problems through functional communication training. *Journal of Applied Behavior Analysis, 18,* 111–126.

Carr, E., & Durand, V. M. (1985). The social-communicative basis of severe behavior problems in children. In S. Reiss & R. Bootzin (Eds.), *Theoretical issues in behavior therapy.* New York: Academic Press.

Coleman, M., & Gillberg, C. (1985). *The biology of the autistic syndrome.* New York: Praeger.

Curcio, F. (1978). Sensorimotor functioning and communication in mute autistic children. *Journal of Autism and Childhood Schizophrenia, 8,* 181–189.

Dawson, G., & Galpert, L. (1986). A developmental model for facilitating the social behavior of autistic children. In E. Schopler & G. Mesibov (Eds.), *Social behavior in autism.* New York: Plenum Press.

Denckla, M. B. (1986). New diagnostic criteria for autism and related behavioral disorders— guidelines for research protocols. *Journal of the American Academy of Child Psychiatry, 25,* 221–224.

Donnellan, A., Mirenda, P., Mesaros, R. A., & Fassbender, L. (1984). Analyzing the communicative functions of aberrant behavior. *Journal of the Association for Persons with Severe Handicaps, 9,* 201–212.

Dore, J. (1986). The development of conversational competence. In R. Scheifelbusch (Ed.), *Language competence: Assessment and intervention.* San Diego: College Hill Press.

Falvey, M. A. (1986). *Community-based curriculum: Instructional strategies for students with severe handicaps.* Baltimore: Paul H. Brookes.

Fay, W. (1979). Personal pronouns and the autistic child. *Journal of Autism and Developmental Disorders, 9,* 247–260.

Fein, D., Pennington, D., Markowitz, P., Braverman, M., & Waterhouse, L. (1986). Toward a neuropsychological model of infantile autism: Are the social deficits primary? *Journal of the American Academy of Child Psychiatry, 25,* 198–212.

Fenske, E. C., Zalenski, S., Krantz, P. J., & McClannahan, L. E. (1985). Age at intervention and treatment outcome for autistic children in a comprehensive intervention program. *Analysis and Intervention in Developmental Disabilities, 5,* 49–58.

Freeman, B. J., & Ritvo, E. R. (1984). The syndrome of autism: Establishing the diagnosis and principles of management. *Pediatric Annals, 13,* 284–296.

Goldstein, H., & Strain, P. (1988). Peers as communication intervention agents: Some new strategies and research findings. *Topics in Language Disorders, 9,* 44–57.

Klinger, L., & Dawson, G. (1992). Facilitating early social and communicative development in children with autism. In S. Warren & J. Reichle (Eds.), *Causes and effects in communication and language intervention* (pp. 157–186) Baltimore: Paul Brookes.

Kurita, H. (1985). Infantile autism with speech loss before the age of thirty months. *Journal of the American Academy of Child Psychiatry, 24,* 191–196.

Lahey, M. (1988). *Language disorders and language development.* New York: Macmillan.

Lord, C. (1985). Autism and the comprehension of language. In E. Schopler & G. Mesibov (Eds.), *Communication problems in autism* (pp. 257–281). New York: Plenum Press.

Lovaas, O. (1977). *The autistic child: Language development through behavior modification.* New York: Wiley.

Lovaas, O. (1981). *Teaching developmentally disabled children. The "Me" book.* Baltimore: University Park Press.

Lovaas, O. I. (1987). Behavioral treatment and normal educational and intellectual functioning in young autistic children. *Journal of Consulting and Clinical Psychology, 55,* 3–9.

MacDonald, J. D. (1985). Language through conversation: A model for intervention with language-delayed persons. In S. Warren & A. Rogers-Warren (Eds.), Teaching functional language: Generalization and maintenance of language skills (pp. 89–122). Baltimore: University Park Press.

MacDonald, J. D. (1989). *Becoming partners with children.* San Antonio, TX: Special Press.

Manolson, A. (1992). *It takes two to talk: Hanen early language guide book* (2nd ed.). Toronto: Hanen Early Language Resource Center.

Marfo, K. (1990). Maternal directiveness in interactions with mentally handicapped children: An analytic commentary. *Journal of Child Psychology and Psychiatry, 31,* 531–549.

Mirenda, P. (1985). Designing pictorial communication systems for physically able-bodied students with severe handicaps. *Augmentative and Alternative Communication, 1,* 58–64.

Mirenda, P., & Schuler, A. (1988). Augmenting communication for persons with autism: Issues and strategies. *Topics in Language Disorders, 9,* 24–43.

Mundy, P., Sigman, M., Ungerer, J. A., & Sherman, T. (1986). Defining the social deficits in autism: The contribution of non-verbal communication measures. *Journal of Child Psychology and Psychiatry, 27,* 657–669.

National Center for Clinical Infant Programs (1985). *Equals in this partnership: Parents of disabled and at-risk infants and toddlers speak to professionals.* Washington, DC: National Maternal and Child Health Clearinghouse.

Owens, R. (1992). *Language development: An introduction* (3rd ed.). Columbus: Merrill Publishing Company.

Powell, T., Hecimovic, A., & Christensen, L. (1992). Meeting the unique needs of families. In D. Berkell (Ed.), *Autism: Identification, education, and treatment* (pp. 187–224). Hillsdale, NJ: Erlbaum.

Powers, M. (1992). Early intervention for children with autism. In D. Berkell (ed.). *Autism: Identification, education, and treatment* (pp. 225–252). Hillsdale, NJ: Erlbaum.

Prizant, B. M. (1982). Part II. Speech-language pathologists and autistic children: What is our role? *Asha Journal, 24,* 531–537.

Prizant, B. M. (1983). Language acquisition and communicative behavior in autism: Toward an understanding of the "whole" of it. *Journal of Speech and Hearing Disorders, 48,* 296–307.

Prizant, B. M. (1987). Clinical implications of echolalic behavior in autism. In T. Layton (Ed.), *Language and treatment of autistic and developmentally disordered children* (pp. 65–88). Springfield, IL: Charles Thomas, Inc.

Prizant, B. M. (1988). Communication in the autistic client. In N. Lass, L. McReynolds, J. Northern, & D. Yoder (Eds.), *Handbook of speech-language pathology and audiology* (pp. 114–139). Philadelphia: B. C. Decker.

Prizant, B. M., & Bailey, D. B. (1992). Facilitating the development of communication skills. In D. B. Bailey & M. Wolery (Eds.), *Teaching infants and preschoolers with handicaps* (pp. 299–361). Columbus, OH: Charles Merrill.

Prizant, B. M., & Meyer, E. C. (in press). Socioemotional aspects of communication disorders in young children and their families. *American Journal of Speech Language Pathology.*

Prizant, B. M. & Rydell, P. (1993). Assessment and intervention strategies for unconventional verbal behavior. In J. Reichle & D. Wacker (Eds.), *Communicative approaches to challenging behavior*. Baltimore: Paul Brookes.

Prizant, B. M., & Schuler, A. (1987a). Facilitating communication: Theoretical foundations. In D. Cohen & A. Donnellan (Eds.), *Handbook of autism and pervasive developmental disorders* (pp. 289–300). New York: Wiley.

Prizant, B. M., & Schuler, A. (1987b). Facilitating communication: Language approaches. In D. Cohen & A. Donnellan (Eds.), *Handbook of autism and pervasive developmental disorders*. New York: Wiley.

Prizant, B. M., & Wetherby, A. M. (1985). Intentional communicative behavior of children with autism: Theoretical and applied issues. *Australian Journal of Human Communication Disorders, 11*, 5–16.

Prizant, B. M., & Wetherby, A. M. (1988). Providing services to children with autism (ages 0 to 2 years) and their families. *Topics in Language Disorders, 9*, 1–23.

Prizant, B. M., & Wetherby, A. M. (1989). Enhancing language and communication in autism: From theory to practice. In G. Dawson (Ed.), *Autism: New perspectives on diagnosis, nature, and treatment* (pp. 282–309). New York: Guilford Press.

Prizant, B. M., & Wetherby, A. M. (1990). Toward an integrated view of early language communication development and socioemotional development. *Topics in Language Disorders, 10*, 1–16.

Prizant, B. M., & Wetherby, A. M. (1993). Communication assessment for young children. *Infants and Young Children, 5*, 20–34.

Quill, K. A. (Ed.). (in press). *Teaching children with autism: Methods to enhance communication and socialization*. Albany, NY: Delmar Publishing Co.

Rossetti, L. (1986). *High-risk infants: Identification, assessment, and intervention*. San Diego: College Hill Press.

Schreibman, L., Koegel, R., Mills, Y. & Burke J. (1984). Training parent–child interactions. In E. Schopler & G. Mesibov (Eds.). *The effects of autism on the family*. New York: Plenum Press.

Schuler, A. L., Peck, C. A., Willard, C. W., & Theimer, K. (1989). Assessment of communicative means and functions through interview: Assessing the communicative abilities of individuals with limited language. *Seminars in Speech and Language, 10*, 51–62.

Schuler, A., & Prizant, B. (1985). Echolalia in autism. In E. Schopler & G. Mesibov (Eds.), *Communication problems in autism*. New York: Plenum Press.

Schuler, A., & Prizant, B. (1987). Facilitating communication: Pre-language approaches. In D. Cohen & A. Donnellan (Eds.), *Handbook of autism and pervasive developmental disorders* (pp. 301–315). New York: Wiley.

Sigman, M., Ungerer, J., Mundy, P., & Sherman, T. (1987). Cognition in autistic children. In D. Cohen & A. Donnellan (Eds.), *Handbook of autism and pervasive developmental disorders*. New York: Wiley.

Smith, M. (1985). Managing the aggressive and self-injurious behavior of adults disabled by autism. *Journal of the Association for Persons with Severe Handicaps, 4*, 228–232.

Snyder-McLean, L., Solomonson, B., McLean, J. E., & Sack, S. (1984). Structuring joint action routines: A strategy for facilitating communication in the classroom. *Seminars in Speech and Language, 5*, 213–228.

Stern, D. (1985). *The interpersonal world of the infant*. New York: Basic Books.

Van Kleeck, A. (1984). Metalinguistic skills: Cutting across spoken and written language and problem solving abilities. In G. Wallach & K. Butler (Eds.), *Language learning disabilities in school-aged children*. Baltimore: Williams & Wilkins.

Watson, L., Lord, C., Schaeffer, B., Schopler, E. (1989). *Teaching spontaneous communication to autistic and developmentally handicapped children*. New York: Irvington Press.

Weitzman, E., & Mayerovitch, J. (1987). *A Pilot Program for the Parents of Young Children with Autism: A Modified Hanen Program.* Unpublished manuscript. Hanen Early Language Resource Centre, Toronto.

Westby, C. (1988). Children's play: Reflections of social competence. *Seminars in Speech and Language, 9,* 1–13.

Wetherby, A. M. (1986). Ontogeny of communicative functions in autism. *Journal of Autism and Developmental Disorders, 16,* 295–316.

Wetherby, A., Cain, D., Yonclas, D., & Walker, V. (1988). Analysis of intentional communication of normal children from the prelinguistic to the multi-word stage. *Journal of Speech and Hearing Research, 31,* 240–252.

Wetherby, A., & Prizant, B. (1989). The expression of communicative intent: Assessment guidelines. *Seminars in Speech and Language, 10,* 77–91.

Wetherby, A. M., & Prizant, B. M. (1992). Profiling young children's communicative competence. In S. Warren & J. Reichle (Eds.), *Causes and effects in communication and language intervention* (pp. 217–253). Baltimore: Paul Brookes.

Wetherby, A. M., & Prizant, B. M. (1993). *Communication and symbolic behavior scales— Normed edition.* Chicago: Riverside Publishing.

Wetherby, A. M., & Prutting, C. (1984). Profiles of communicative and cognitive-social abilities in autistic children. *Journal of Speech and Hearing Research, 27,* 364–377.

Wetherby, A. M., Yonclas, D., & Bryan, A. (1989). Communicative profiles of handicapped preschool children: Implications for early identification. *Journal of Speech and Hearing Disorders, 54,* 148–158.

6

Behavior Management in the Preschool Years

MARY E. VAN BOURGONDIEN

INTRODUCTION

The preschool years are a time of great change in the lives of normally developing youngsters. During this time of rapid development, parents report a number of common problems related to toilet training, fears, sleeping, bad habits, noncompliance, and aggression (Schroeder, Gordon, & Hawk, 1983). It comes as no surprise that children with autism exhibit similar sorts of behavior difficulties which tend to be exacerbated by the social, cognitive, and language deficits that characterize this disorder. In addition, they exhibit behavior problems, such as poor play skills and lack of initiative, more directly related to their specific handicap.

In DeMeyer's (1979) in-depth study of 58 children with autism, she reported that parents found the preschool years to be the most difficult time for them and for their children. Seventy-eight percent of these children had the greatest difficulties in the areas of speech, social relations and general disposition between 2 and 4 years of age. DeMeyer speculated that these years are particularly difficult because it is a time when parental fears, anxieties, and feelings of helplessness

MARY E. VAN BOURGONDIEN • Division TEACCH, Department of Psychiatry, University of North Carolina at Chapel Hill, Chapel Hill, North Carolina 27599-7180.

Preschool Issues in Autism, edited by Eric Schopler *et al.* Plenum Press, New York, 1993.

are at a peak. Generally, this is the age when parents first learn about their child's difficulty and struggle to find out what it will mean to their child and family. Given the tremendous developmental progress that normally developing children make during this time, the developmental difficulties that children with autism display appear quite dramatic in contrast.

This chapter will review the types of problems seen in autism and will describe how these problems relate to both normal development and the underlying deficits of autism. Ways of preventing behavior problems through structured teaching techniques and working with families will be presented along with a strategy for analyzing and problem-solving around specific behavior problems.

The information provided in this chapter is derived from the research and clinical experience of the TEACCH program in North Carolina.

SPECIFIC BEHAVIOR PROBLEMS

In an informal survey of parental concerns, the clinical staff at TEACCH have noted that the primary behavioral difficulties presented by families of young children are aggression, lack of response to discipline, eating problems, poor play skills, lack of initiative, sleep problems, temper tantrums, and toileting difficulties. These behavior problems have been conceptualized as being the overt signs of an underlying deficit related to autism (Schopler, 1989). For example, Figure 6-1 depicts an iceberg where above the surface are the visible behaviors of lack of response to spanking, scolding, isolation, or guilt induction. Below the water line are listed some of the hypotheses as to why an autistic child may not be responding to a given discipline technique. For example, "time out" or isolating an autistic child from his or her surroundings may not be effective because the child's social deficits make being alone preferable. Through careful assessment, the most likely explanation for a behavior in a given child can be identified and used to develop an appropriate intervention strategy. In the case of discipline problems, most children with autism respond best if the behavior problem can be prevented from occurring in the first place rather than trying to discipline the child after the fact.

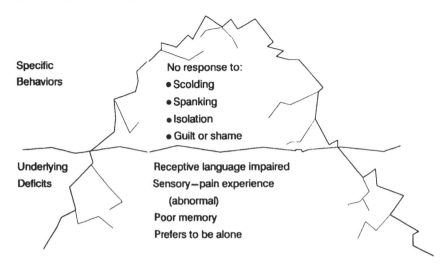

Specific
Behaviors

No response to:
● Scolding
● Spanking
● Isolation
● Guilt or shame

Underlying
Deficits

Receptive language impaired
Sensory–pain experience
(abnormal)
Poor memory
Prefers to be alone

Fig. 6-1. Discipline.

Aggression

Among the most frequent parental concerns is the occurrence of physical aggression in children with autism. Aggression toward others can include pushing, hitting, spitting, biting, or throwing things. Konstantareas and Homatidis (1989) reported such aggressive acts in 13 out of 44 autistic children ages 2 to 12.

Normally developing children also often display physical aggression. However, this physical aggression gradually gives way to verbal aggression between the ages of 2 and 6 years (Schroeder et al., 1983). The aggression usually is used as a means of gaining possession of a lost or desired plaything. The decrease in aggression after age 6 is generally associated with increased cognitive abilities that allow children to evaluate the consequences of their actions and to develop alternate solutions. This ability to generate alternate solutions is lacking in children with social handicaps (Spivak & Shure, 1974).

Aggression in children with autism is frequently related to their frustration over their inability to communicate. They have difficulty understanding what is expected of them as well as in communicating their needs to others. Sensory misconceptions and the lack of awareness of their own or other's feelings can prevent them from learning the consequences of their aggressive actions. Poor social judgment interferes with their ability to generate alternate solutions that enable other children to develop more adaptive coping strategies.

The primary approach to reducing aggressive behavior in preschoolers with autism is to increase their understanding of their environment through the use of predictable routines or visual cues. Our assumption in most instances is that children are aggressive because of confusion about what to expect or frustration over their inability to express themselves. For example, one might find that a preschooler begins to get aggressive when one activity is ending and it is time to do something else. By giving the child a way to anticipate what is coming next, such as showing a ball to indicate it's time to go outside, the child's confusion and subsequent aggressive behavior is likely to diminish.

Noncompliance and Discipline Problems

The second most frequent concern reported by parents in the TEACCH program is noncompliance or a lack of response to discipline. Techniques frequently used with other children such as scolding, spanking, isolation, or guilt induction are not as effective.

The preschool years between ages 2 and 4 are typically when noncompliance is at its peak in normally developing children due to the pressures of socialization and routinization (Schroeder et al., 1983).

In preschoolers with autism, the typical lack of response to parental commands is exacerbated by the children's difficulty understanding what is being asked. In some cases their inability to perform the behavior being asked of them further complicates the situation. Their subsequent lack of response to verbal discipline techniques, such as scolding or shaming, is often due to their impaired understanding of language or to poor memory. Spankings fail to produce the desired effect partially because of these same cognitive factors but also because the sense of pain in children with autism may be atypical or nonexistent. Perhaps the most common discipline technique is "time out" or removal of the child from a socially reinforcing situation. For those who prefer to be alone and find social experiences overwhelming or unpleasant, time out techniques designed to decrease behavior may actually reinforce it.

As mentioned previously, the best way to manage discipline problems in preschoolers with autism is to prevent the problem from happening in the first place. Sometimes this means avoiding situations that the child is not yet ready to handle, e.g., long waits in restaurants. In other situations it will require setting up visual cues and physical structure to help the child know what is expected.

Eating

Eating problems are among the most frustrating difficulties encountered by parents of preschoolers with autism (DeMeyer, 1979). Fifty-nine percent of parents of normally developing youngsters report a number of feeding problems during these years, while 94% of parents of children with autism report difficulties with feeding (DeMeyer, 1979). Most children develop specific likes and dislikes at age 3 (Schaffer & Millman, 1981); the autistic child's rigid preferences or refusal to try new foods takes this behavior to an extreme. Problems with chewing are frequently reported. Pica, eating inedible substances such as clay, dirt, plaster, or paint, is also common, and tends to occur most often between the ages of 1 and 3 (Schaffer & Millman, 1981).

Again, behaviors typical of many toddlers and preschoolers are exacerbated by autism. Poor food recognition and impaired sensory taste perception may affect the ability of autistic children to perceive the differences between edible and inedible substances. An impaired hunger drive may make food less appealing. A resistance to change and insistence on sameness may make it very difficult to introduce new varieties or textures of food.

Some parents have successfully dealt with difficulties with chewing or with textures by using a blender to puree a wide variety of food. By gradually increasing the amount of texture, the child can be introduced to a wider variety of foods. Others have found that new foods can be introduced if the meal involves a routine of eating a new food followed by a more familiar item. One parent of a toddler who had a tendency to pick up anything and everything from the floor and put it in his mouth found that hanging a pacifier around his neck where he could always find it solved the problem.

Poor Play Skills

In the typical child, there is a progression from solitary to parallel play at around age 2, to cooperative play with one other child at age 3, and to cooperative play in groups at age 5 (Parten, 1932). The desire for interactions with peers is great (Manosevitz, Prentice, & Wilson, 1973). The play of preschool children includes the ability to use their imaginations and to engage in pretend play.

Children with autism, however, are generally not able to amuse themselves, use toys appropriately, or play with others. They may break toys or play with them in some atypical or repetitive fashion, such as lining them up or just spinning small parts. Underlying these behaviors are deficits in language and imaginary play. These children's organizational deficits make it very difficult for them to organize their time by initiating and sustaining more appropriate play activities. As they get older, they do not understand the concepts of sharing or taking turns or the rules of specific games that enable other children to play cooperatively.

A first step in teaching young children play skills is to set up a structured teaching situation to teach the child what toy to play with, how to use the toy, and how to know when they are finished. Many toys for young children do not have a clear use and it's hard for children with autism to know how to use them or when they are finished. Puzzles and shape boxes are often the toys they do best with because they are intrinsically structured with clear beginnings and ends. Dolls and toy cars are more difficult because their use is not concretely defined, and they do not have a clear ending point. They require children to create a function and to know when they are finished. Establishing "work" sessions to teach play skills might involve sitting a child at a table with the toys he or she is to use in baskets sequenced from left to right, with a larger basket for completed activities at the far right. The use of the baskets helps children know what toys to play with, how many toys they will play with, and when they are finished. Starting with the more structured toys will help children learn the system before introducing toys that are more open-ended. For the more open-ended toys such as dolls and dollhouses, children often benefit from being taught concrete routines for using these materials. Once children learn to use these materials in the more structured teaching situations, the next step is to help them learn to use these materials in a play area.

One parent of a preschooler found that when she took her child to the park and said "go play," instead of going to the swings or slide, he ran around flapping his arms. She decided that the underlying problem was that her son did not understand the words "go play." So each day she took him to the park, said "go play," and then took him to the slide or swings. Eventually, all she had to say as they got out of the car was "go play" and her son ran to the equipment to play.

Lack of Initiative

The lack of initiative and frequently extreme dependence on external cues is a source of concern for parents of children with autism of all ages. These children can appear to be lazy or unmotivated as they wait for others to provide prompts or cues in order to initiate or sustain an activity.

This lack of initiative is frequently related to the inability to organize and sequence behavior. Further complicating the issue can be a low arousal level, a poor concept of time, and a lack of understanding of future rewards. These concepts that help develop motivation in normally developing preschoolers are lacking in many young children with autism. Again their social deficits reduce the effectiveness of many typical sources of motivation such as pleasing others or social praise.

Initiating appropriate play activities is a frequent issue even after a child has learned in more structured situations how to play with specific materials. The process of choosing play materials can be facilitated by having a board with pictures of familiar free time activities from which the child can choose or a bookcase where the available options are individually displayed and organized for the child to use.

Sleep Problems

In a study of 44 children with autism, Konstantareas and Homatidis (1989) found sleep problems to be the most common problem reported by parents (70%). Many typical preschoolers experience transitory problems with sleep at different ages. Resistance to sleep and waking are the most frequently reported sleep difficulties in normally developing 2 to 3 year olds (Schroeder *et al.*, 1983). However, their problems usually are mild compared to those of children with autism (DeMeyer, 1979). In addition to more frequent problems with falling asleep and nighttime awakenings, parents of autistic children report concerns about wandering at night (DeMeyer, 1979).

These sleep difficulties are believed to be related to the hyperactivity and distractibility observed in many children with this disorder. A resistance to change can make going to bed a difficult time, and hypersensitivity to noise can cause problems with falling and staying asleep.

Increased physical exercise during the day can help increase the likelihood that the child will sleep at night. Having a predictable bedtime routine with calming activities (e.g., a bath) just before bed can make the transition go more smoothly. One parent found that by putting a rocking chair and music (two things her son really liked) in his room, she was able to establish a routine where he sat in the chair and listened to the music until he became drowsy. Slowly he learned to make the transition to bed himself when he became sleepy.

Putting a bell on the child's door or continuing to use a baby monitor can help parents be aware of the child's nighttime activities. Others have found that a wooden baby gate or dutch doors have helped keep the child from wandering at night.

Tantrums

Temper tantrums are observed most frequently in children between the ages of 2 and 4 and seem to occur most often when children are tired and frustrated. In a sample of 44 children with autism, almost 30% displayed self-injurious behaviors (Konstantareas & Homatidis, 1989). Screaming without apparent cause and destroying toys or other materials are other forms of tantrums noted in children with autism.

These tantrums are frequently due to children with autism's tendencies to get easily frustrated and their impaired ability to communicate their needs to other people. Their unstable emotional responsivity may increase the likelihood of their becoming enraged. Hypersensitivity to even subtle changes in their environment or their parents' responses also may increase the likelihood of the autistic youngster to engage in temper tantrums.

As with aggression and noncompliance, the most successful approach to dealing with tantrums is to carefully analyze the situation in which they are occurring to determine what aspect of the situation may be confusing or frustrating to the child with autism. Generally, adding routines and visual cues to help the child predict what will happen next are part of the solution.

Toileting

In order to be toilet trained, a child must be able to voluntarily control the sphincter muscles, communicate needs verbally or nonverbally, and be motivated to control the impulse to defecate and urinate (Leventhal, 1981). To be successful, they need to plan, organize, and execute the many sequences involved in toileting and hygiene. Most children are toilet trained by the age of 4 years, except for bedwetting in boys (Routh, 1980).

Problems with wetting and soiling are a frequent problem in children with autism (Konstantareas & Homatidis, 1989). They may also smear feces, a behavior more typically characteristic of 15- to 21-month-old-children at the end of their naps. Eliminating in the wrong place, such as out in the yard or behind the living room curtains, is also reported. Communication handicaps, impaired organization of the toileting sequence, poor sequential memory, a tendency to get distracted, and a lack of recognition of body signals all can make it difficult for an autistic child to become toilet trained or get to the toilet in time once trained. Children who have learned to urinate or defecate in one place (e.g., diapers or a potty seat) may have difficulty changing to the toilet. Again, the motivators that usually work with other children ("big boy" underwear or the desire to please) are not as effective in training children with autism.

One of the most basic approaches to teaching toileting skills is to develop a routine time for the child to sit on the toilet or potty seat. It is best to select times when the child is most likely to need to go; often this is right after meals and when awakening in the morning and going to bed at night. By pairing the trip to the bathroom with a specific object, such as toilet paper, the less verbal youngster begins to understand where he or she is going and what will happen there.

WORKING WITH FAMILIES

An essential ingredient in managing the behavior of autistic children is the involvement of parents in the treatment of their child. Collaboration between parents and professionals is instrumental in the prevention of behavior problems in children with autism (Schopler, 1976, 1978). Parents as cotherapists provide information about what makes their child unique, while the professional shares information about autism (Schopler, Mesibov, Shigley, & Bashford, 1984). The mutual support between parent and professional helps them both cope with the frustrations that can occur when treating children with severe developmental disabilities. Together they advocate the needs of the child in the larger community.

The research has shown that parent training improves the skills and behaviors of the child with autism (Marcus, Lansing, Andrews, & Schopler, 1978; Short, 1984). In addition, the collaboration between parents and professionals in a community-based program has led to a significant decrease in the number of children requiring institutionalization (Schopler, Mesibov, & Baker, 1982; Schopler, 1989).

PREVENTION OF BEHAVIOR PROBLEMS
THROUGH STRUCTURED TEACHING

Parents of toddlers and preschoolers quickly learn that the most effective means of dealing with many of these challenging behaviors is to prevent them from occurring in the first place through household engineering (Ilg, Ames, & Baker, 1981). For normally developing youngsters this means having appropriate expectations, limiting situations they cannot handle such as long waits, or moving things out of their reach to avoid having to constantly say "don't touch." Judiciously placed naps or snack times can substantially reduce behavior problems associated with fatigue or hunger.

For the parents of children with autism, restructuring the environment also means finding ways to compensate for the underlying deficits that contribute to the behavior. The most pervasive of these difficulties is the impaired ability to communicate. Inability to understand what others are saying and difficulties with organization and sequential memory make it hard for these children to know what is expected of them in the immediate or near future. Difficulties understanding the concepts of time and future rewards interfere with learning many of the skills taught during these early years. Their distractibility and tendency to become easily frustrated are factors that also need to be considered in structuring an optimal learning environment.

The techniques that have proven effective for structuring classrooms are equally appropriate for restructuring the home setting (Landrus & Mesibov, 1986; Schopler, 1989; Schopler, Brehm, Kinsbourne, & Reichler, 1971). Based on an individualized assessment of the child, the goal is to change the environment so that developmentally appropriate expectations are communicated to the child through routines and the use of visual cues. The development of adaptive routines around eating, sleeping, dressing, and other daily events can improve children's understanding of what is going to happen next as well as their willingness to comply. Visual cues are usually the best to use because visual perception skills are generally better developed than language skills and because visual aids are concrete and do not require memory. Visual cues can take the forms of physical structure, a daily schedule, work systems, or materials structures (Landrus & Mesibov, 1986; Schopler, 1989).

Physical Structure

Physical structure refers to the way the classroom or household is set up or organized. The placement of furniture and materials can communicate the function of a particular space. Clear boundaries can help children know where they are supposed to be and what the expectations are for them in that area. For example, a fence around an outdoor play area or a rug in the family room can help a child learn not to stray while dinner is being prepared. Auditory and visual distractions should be limited in areas where new skills are being taught. For example, having a music box on in a play area may be fine, but during mealtime when table skills are being taught, a TV or radio may distract the child from the task at hand. The materials that the teacher or parent is going to use with the child with autism should be placed in an appropriate place and labeled so that they are easily accessible.

Daily Schedule

A daily schedule tells in a visual way what will happen next and the sequence of the day's activities. For children who have difficulty understanding what others are telling them and who cannot remember sequences, a visual schedule reduces confusion and helps them learn to anticipate where to go next.

The most basic schedule is an object system where a child is given an object to indicate where they are to go next. Giving a child a coat indicates it is time to go outside; giving a roll of toilet paper indicates it is time to go to the bathroom. The child can carry the object as a constant reminder of where he or she is going.

For children who understand pictures, a posted picture schedule can provide information about where to go next, what will happen there, and the sequence of the day's activities. Depending on the needs and skills of the individual, the pictures can be either photographs or line drawings. Children who need a reminder of where they are going when moving from one place to another can carry the picture with them and match it to a corresponding picture when they arrive at their destination.

For those children not able to absorb lots of information at one time, the schedule can be for part of a day. For those who need to know the entire sequence of events in order to feel comfortable, it can be for a full day. The full-day schedule is particularly helpful for indicating the occurrence of special events that are not part of the usual routine.

For youngsters with a sight-word vocabulary, pictures can be paired with words to make a combination of a picture and written schedule. As a child understands more words, the schedule can be entirely written.

Regardless of the type of visual cue, all of the schedules can help decrease confusion and help children with autism understand what is going to happen next. Any of these visual cues can be used to help make transitions or they can stay in one place depending on the memory and organizational skills of the child.

Work System

The daily schedule directs children where to go next; the work system tells them what to do when they get there. Ideally the work system tells preschool students what work to do, how much work to do, when they are finished, and what the reinforcement will be. In the most basic work system, the child's work is placed on the left in separate containers, the reward is visible, and there is a finished box on the right where completed work is placed. The children can see the work that needs to be completed, they can tell the number of tasks by the number of baskets, and they know they are finished when all the baskets from their left are gone and placed in the finished box on their right. Receiving the reinforcer at the end of the task(s) further helps to define the concept of what is finished and what will happen next.

A more flexible work system or "to do" list is a list of color cards. A child takes the first card, matches it to a work box of the same color, does the work, and then places it in the finished bin. The number of color cards indicates the number of tasks and the order of cards from top to bottom or left to right denotes the sequence. Depending on the child's organizational skills and mobility, the work boxes can be in reach of the seat or placed on a bookshelf away from the desk. The reward or picture of the reward should be placed to indicate where in the sequence it is received. Some children may need a reinforcer after every task, while others may be able to wait until after three tasks are completed. The reinforcer or motivator will vary from child to child. Completing work and being able to go to a free-time area is a sufficient motivator for some children, while an edible or the opportunity to have a special object will be needed for others. For children with more cognitive skills, the color list can be replaced by a list of letters, numbers, or words that correspond to the work tasks. In all instances, work systems visually inform students what work to complete, what sequence to follow, and what the reinforcer will be. The system is individualized by the degree of mobility required of the student to get the work and by the kind and frequency of the reinforcer.

Task Organization or Material Structure

The work system visually indicates what work a student is to do but does not show how to do it. In order to complete tasks, students need visual cues or directions. Establishing a predictable routine around bedtime, mealtime, toileting, bathing, or any other task can help children learn to complete tasks with increasing independence.

Organizing necessary materials helps children function more independently. Giving only the materials needed for the specific task and placing the materials in containers will keep them from being scattered around the work area.

Picture representations such as jigs can help children complete tasks without having to understand verbal directions. These can include picture lists for gathering materials or a picture sequence indicating how materials are to be assembled. For children who read, written lists and directions may be more effective than verbal instructions.

PROBLEM SOLVING AROUND BEHAVIOR DIFFICULTIES

Most behavior difficulties associated with autism can be managed by understanding how a behavior relates to the central characteristics of autism and then modifying the environment in order to clarify expectations and compensate for areas of deficit. If a behavior problem persists, a more intensive study of the difficulty may be required. The following discussion describes the procedures used by the professionals at TEACCH to develop an individualized behavior management plan (Division TEACCH Summer Training, 1990).

The first step in dealing with any behavior problem is to define the behavior in objective, concrete language. The description should be so clear and objective that even a newcomer can determine when the behavior occurs.

The next step is to determine the history of the behavior. How long has it been happening? Is it a new behavior? Is it changing? Is it getting better or worse? The data collected about the occurrence of the behavior includes information about the frequency of the behavior and its antecedents and consequences. What seems to set off the behavior? When, where, and with whom does it occur? What does the child do just before the behavior occurs? What happens afterward? What do the parents or teachers do? What does the child do? How does the behavior affect the child's environment—family, school or neighborhood?

Before proceeding any further, a decision needs to be made about the importance of changing the behavior. This decision will be based on the assessment of whether or not the behavior is interfering with the child's learning or other children's learning. If the behavior is disruptive to others or is dangerous, there is good reason to change it. Behaviors that are unusual but do not present any difficulty to the child or others, or are of low frequency, may not be worth pursuing depending on other priorities.

Before developing a plan for managing the behavior, it is important to try to determine why it occurs. The behavior data collected is reviewed to determine if there is any pattern to when, where, and with whom the behavior occurs. Commonality in the types of settings or expectations that seem to set off the behavior are explored. By taking the child's point of view, it is possible to make some guesses about reasons for the behavior. Things that may be confusing or that the child may not understand need to be explored.

In addition to the behavioral data, a review of the child's developmental level is an essential part of problem solving. It is necessary to determine what the child understands and can or cannot do, remembering that what an autistic child does in one area of development or in one setting may not be predictive of what that child can do in a different area. In reviewing the hypotheses regarding the reasons for the behavior problem, whether the child has the understanding or the skills to be successful is examined.

Based on this careful assessment, a plan for managing the behavior in one situation in which it occurs is developed. Depending on the hypotheses developed about why the behavior is occurring, the plan will include ways of clarifying the expectations for the child, and lessening the confusion. Efforts to prevent the behavior from occurring such as altering the environment to increase the child's understanding or changing expectations to match his or her developmental ability will be pursued. Positive reinforcement for behaviors that are incompatible with the problem behavior may be added, keeping in mind that the types of things that are reinforcing and motivating to children with autism are often very different from things other children may find rewarding.

Depending on the nature and severity of the behavior, it may be necessary to choose a meaningful way to let the child know that the behavior is not appropriate. Exactly how one says "no" to the behavior will depend on what has already been tried, and the individual child's learning style.

This problem-solving approach can be applied to any of the common behavioral difficulties of preschool children. Let's use as an example a 4-year-old boy with autism who defecates in his pants while playing outside every afternoon. A review of his toileting history indicates that he has never had bowel movements in the toilet. He had started to use a potty seat that was placed in his bedroom, but when this was removed to encourage him to use the toilet he resumed soiling his pants. He has one bowel movement a day, usually in the afternoon. Changing this behavior is very important to his parents, who have two younger children. In reviewing the data, it appears as if the child knows when he has to defecate but is confused about the appropriate place. Now he appears to wait until he's outside to defecate. He initially seemed to make good progress when the potty seat was used. In order to clarify expectations about where to have bowel movements, the parents reinitiated the use of the potty seat, but moved it to the bathroom. They built into the child's daily routine times to sit on the potty seat. They chose these times based on catching him when he was most likely to have a bowel movement, right after lunch and before going outside to play. While the boy was sitting on the potty seat, he was given a special toy to hold. He only got to have this toy while he was sitting in the bathroom. This favorite toy was used to communicate to the boy that he was doing the right thing and to help relax him so he would be successful. If he had a bowel movement on the potty, he was given a treat when he was finished. Within a short time after initiating this approach, the soiling stopped.

The preschool years are a challenging time for all parents. The typical problems that arise during this time of rapid development are exacerbated by the characteristics of autism. In addition to understanding the typical course of these behaviors, it is important for parents and teachers to understand how the characteristics of autism affect the child's behavior. This understanding can facilitate the structuring of the environment in order to increase the child's understanding of expectations and to help compensate for skills the child does not currently have.

REFERENCES

DeMeyer, M. K. (1979). *Parents and children in autism.* New York: Wiley.

Division TEACCH Summer Training. (1990). *Problem solving approach to behavior management.* Unpublished manuscript, University of North Carolina at Chapel Hill, Division TEACCH, Chapel Hill.

Ilg, F. L., Ames, L. B., & Baker, S. M. (1981). *Child behavior.* New York: Harper & Row.

Konstantareas, M. M., & Homatidis, S. (1989). Assessing child symptom severity and stress in parents of autistic children. *Journal of Child Psychology and Psychiatry, 30,* 459–470.

Landrus, R., & Mesibov, G. B. (1986). *Structured teaching.* Unpublished manuscript, University of North Carolina at Chapel Hill, Division TEACCH, Chapel Hill.

Leventhal, J. M. (1981). Enuresis. In S. Gabel (Ed.), *Behavior problems of childhood* (pp. 195–211). New York: Grune & Stratton.

Manosevitz, M., Prentice, N. M., & Wilson, F. (1973). Individual and family correlates of imaginary companions in preschool children. *Developmental Psychology, 8,* 72–79.

Marcus, L., Lansing, M., Andrews, C., & Schopler, E. (1978). Improvement of teaching effectiveness in parents of autistic children. *Journal of the American Academy of Child Psychiatry, 17,* 625–639.

Parten, M. B. (1932). Social participation among preschool children. *Journal of Abnormal and Social Psychology, 27,* 243–269.

Routh, D. K. (1980). The preschool child. In S. Gabel & M. T. Erickson (Eds.), *Child development and developmental disabilities* (pp. 21–42). Boston: Little, Brown.

Schaffer, C. E., & Millman, H. L. (1981). *How to help children with common problems.* New York: Plenum Press.

Schopler, E. (1976). Towards reducing behavior problems in autistic children. In L. Wing (Ed.), *Early childhood autism* (2nd ed.) (pp. 221–245). Oxford: Pergamon Press.

Schopler, E. (1978). Prevention of psychosis through alternate education. In S. J. Apter (Ed.), *Focus on prevention* (pp. 79–94). New York: Syracuse University Press.

Schopler, E. (1989). Principles for directing both education, treatment and research. In C. Gillberg (Ed.), *Diagnosis and treatment of autism* (pp. 167–183). New York: Plenum Press.

Schopler, E., Brehm, S. S., Kinsbourne, M., & Reichler, R. J. (1971). Effect of treatment structure on development in autistic children. *Archives of General Psychiatry, 24,* 415–421.

Schopler, E., Mesibov, G. B., & Baker, A. (1982). Evaluation of treatment for autistic children and their parents. *Journal of the American Academy of Child Psychiatry, 21,* 262–267.

Schopler, E., Mesibov, G. B., Shigley, H., & Bashford, A. (1984). Helping autistic children through their parents: The TEACCH model. In E. Schopler & G. B. Mesibov (Eds.), *The effects of autism on the family* (pp. 65–81). New York: Plenum Press.

Schroeder, C. S., Gordon, B. N., & Hawk, B. (1983). Clinical problems of the preschool child. In C. E. Walker & M. C. Roberts (Eds.), *Handbook of Clinical Child Psychology* (pp. 296–334). New York: Wiley.

Short, A. (1984). Short-term treatment outcome using parents as co-therapists for their own autistic children. *Journal of Child Psychology and Psychiatry and Allied Disciplines, 25,* 443–458.

Spivack, G., & Shure, M. B. (1974). *Social adjustment of young children: A cognitive approach to solving real-life problems.* San Francisco: Jossey-Bass.

III

Diagnostic, Assessment,
and Programmatic Aspects

7

Assessment of the Young Autistic Child

LEE M. MARCUS and WENDY L. STONE

INTRODUCTION

This chapter will cover issues and methods in the assessment of preschoolers with autism and related severe disorders of communication.
Aspects of diagnosis will be reviewed as a backdrop to a review of
behavioral characteristics using the current DSM-III-R (American Psychiatric Association, 1987) symptom clusters as a basis to describe
empirical data and implications for clinical approaches. Following a
discussion of general issues in assessment, including how both diagnosis and assessment differ between the young preschooler and the older
autistic child, the final section will discuss the relationship between
assessment and treatment planning.

DIAGNOSIS AND THE PRESCHOOLER

The syndrome of autism, originally described by Kanner (1943),
has been recognized as an enduring and empirically determined psychiatric diagnostic label (Schopler, 1983). Over the years, the definition
and description have been refined and modified in the light of research
findings (Rutter, 1978). These changes have resulted in a consensus

LEE M. MARCUS • Division TEACCH, Department of Psychiatry, University of North Carolina
at Chapel Hill, Chapel Hill, North Carolina 27599-7180   WENDY L. STONE • Department of
Pediatrics, Vanderbilt University School of Medicine, Nashville, Tennessee 37203.

Preschool Issues in Autism, edited by Eric Schopler *et al.* Plenum Press, New York, 1993.

that the major criteria include impairments in social relatedness, delayed and deviant language development and communication, and restricted and repetitive interests and behaviors.

DSM-III (American Psychiatric Association, 1980) included autism for the first time under a new classification, pervasive developmental disorders (PDD), which had categories for infantile autism, child onset pervasive developmental disorder (COPDD), and residual categories for milder cases or for those no longer meeting all the criteria. There were a number of problems with the DSM-III system: COPDD seemed merely a variation of autism with a later age of onset and looser criteria; infantile autism was too strictly defined and over-emphasized speech rather than basic communicative deficits; and there was a de-emphasis on autism in adulthood by allowing for the use of the "residual" category.

DSM-III-R (American Psychiatric Association, 1987) has simplified the PDD classification and has provided highly specific behavioral descriptors that have a developmental orientation and are intended to cover the entire age and intelligence spectrum. Simplification was achieved by reducing the classification to two categories: autistic disorder (AD) and pervasive developmental disorder not otherwise specified (PDDNOS). Both categories include the three major areas listed above. AD is diagnosed if, from a possible total of 16 behaviorally defined characteristics, at least 8 are indicated with a minimum of 2 from the social area and 1 from the other two areas. PDDNOS is applied to any other cases not meeting this standard. While this is an improvement over DSM-III in terms of precision, having a developmental focus and a more empirical basis, further research is needed to establish the reliability and validity of the revised system.

Although the diagnosis of autism has traditionally and typically been associated with the early school years (ages 5 to 6), the recent increase in professional and public awareness has resulted in younger children being identified. Within the TEACCH program in North Carolina (Schopler, 1987), over the past few years, the number of children under the age of 5 referred for evaluation has doubled while the rate of referrals for school-age children has remained constant. Although professionals are better able to recognize the early signs of possible autism, there remains some reluctance to apply the diagnosis to very young children. One clinical reason seems to be a concern over alarming parents unnecessarily or somehow interfering with the child's chance for successful development by premature labeling.

Another, perhaps more cogent reason is that the diagnosis is more ambiguous in preschoolers than at later ages. The diagnostic process with the preschooler differs in some respects from that with the older autistic child. The differentiation from mental retardation and language disorders without autism is somewhat more difficult to make. There is a greater overlap at the younger ages and less obvious discrepancies between global development and language and communication and social delays and deviances. There is a tendency for language and social development, two of the defining features of autism, to covary, and if there is not yet an easily recognized pattern of ritualistic or stereotypic behaviors, the autistic syndrome may not be obvious. On the other hand, autistic characteristics, especially lack of social relatedness, can be very dramatic, more so than with the older child whose social interests tend to improve (Mesibov, 1983).

Despite the potential ambiguity, there are far more advantages than disadvantages to early diagnosis. First, having a clearcut label helps the family understand and gain control over their situation. Rarely, in our experience, do parents consider this diagnostic statement a disservice, even though, of course, such news is always unsettling and often a shock. Instead, it is usually received with some relief that there is an explanation for their child's puzzling behaviors and learning patterns and hope that with the diagnosis can come specific treatment. Definitive diagnosis avoids the confusion of vague labels (e.g., communication-disordered with autistic features), uncertainties which force the parents to seek further evaluations, and inevitable delays of appropriate services when nonspecific terminology is given. The major advantage of a clear diagnosis is the ability to plan an effective intervention based on the principles of structure, individualization, parental involvement, emphasis on socialization and communication training, and the development of independence in learning and behavior patterns so critical for future success. Delaying the diagnosis may mean encouraging nondirective, open-ended, child-as-self-directed learner approaches, adequate for most normal and many mildly handicapped youngsters, but ineffective for the vast majority of autistic children.

Can an early diagnosis ever be harmful? A problem can arise if the label of autism causes the clinician to miss other conditions such as mental retardation or deafness. Given the potential misconception that autism and mental retardation are mutually exclusive, the clinician must guard against assuming that a diagnosis of autism means that the child has normal intellectual potential. It is also important that parents recognize that having autism is not somehow more favorable than having mental retardation. A second problem might occur if the diagnosis fails to lead to an individualized treatment program, based on a careful and comprehensive assessment, and/or if reassessments are not periodically carried out, allowing the child to be placed in an inappropriate educational and treatment "track." If the diagnosis becomes an end in itself, it can lead to frustration and stagnation in the treatment process. However, it is not diagnosis per se that is at fault, but the failure to move beyond this initial step. As will be discussed later, research is beginning to highlight early developmental precursors to autism such as imitation, which may prove to discriminate more reliably than symbolic toy play among younger children (Stone, Lemanek, Fishel, Fernandez, & Altemeier, 1990).

A final issue for consideration in early diagnosis are the variations in the course of development within the first 3 years (DeMyer, 1979; Watson & Marcus, 1988). Although by age 3 the main features of autism are usually manifested (Volkmar, Cohen, & Paul, 1986), there appear to be several possible developmental sequences: generally slow development across all areas with increasingly differentiated symptoms of communication and relatedness; fairly normal development until 18–24 months, then marked regression or at least failure to continue to develop normally; or normal development for a year and then a gradual falling off. Being aware of these differing developmental sequences can help the clinician detect significant early signs. In addition, parents can benefit from the knowledge that their child's seemingly paradoxical behavior (e.g., loss of a 20–30 word vocabulary) is fairly common in young autistic children.

At this point, the distinction between diagnosis and assessment should be made. Diagnosis refers to those features of the child shared by others, resulting in the classification of autism, whereas assessment provides detailed information about skill levels, learning styles, patterns of strengths and weaknesses, and potential for successful treatment and adaptation. While diagnosis deals essentially with the commonality among characteristics, assessment emphasizes the unique qualities of individuals. Given this distinction, the potential problems in the diagnostic process of ambiguity, developmental variation, and vagueness in labeling become less relevant if the specific learning patterns and behavioral characteristics are clearly identified.

CHARACTERISTICS OF YOUNG AUTISTIC CHILDREN

This section will present a review of the behavioral characteristics of young autistic children. Although preschool-aged children must meet the same general set of diagnostic criteria as older children with autism, developmental changes in the expression of specific features of autism have been reported by many investigators (e.g., Volkmar & Cohen, 1988; Wing, 1988). In keeping with the theme of this book, the present review will therefore be restricted to empirical studies that have focused on preschool children. The behavioral categories reviewed correspond to the primary diagnostic characteristics of DSM-III-R: social behavior, communication, and activities and interests. Studies employing parent report measures as well as observational or experimental procedures are included. Characteristics of the studies are presented in Table 7-1.

Social Behavior

The category of social behavior includes three broad areas of social functioning: relating to adults, interacting with peers, and imitating the actions of others.

Relating to Adults

This area of social behavior has received the most research attention; it encompasses behaviors indicative of social awareness and interest, interpersonal involvement, and attachment. The majority of parents of young autistic children describe severe deficits in their children's social awareness and relating. As many as 85% to 96% of parents report that their children ignore people or "look through" people as if they were not there (Volkmar, Cohen, & Paul, 1986). Difficulty forming interpersonal relationships is reported more frequently for young

Table 7-1. Empirical Research
Focusing on Characteristics of Young Autistic Children

Authors	Date	Subjects	Ages	Characteristic(s) studied
Observational/Experimental Studies				
Dawson & Adams	1984	15 AUT	49–80 mos	S
DeMyer et al.	1972	12 AUT/SCZ	42–83 mos	S
		5 MR	46–99 mos	
Mundy et al.	1986	18 AUT	$M = 53.3$ mos	C, A
		18 MR	$M = 50.2$ mos[a]	
		18 NOR	$M = 22.2$ mos[a]	
Shapiro et al.	1987	15 AUT	25–59 mos	S
		10 APDD	34–56 mos	
		3 MR	38–63 mos	
		8 DLD	30–45 mos	
Sherman et al.	1983	16 AUT	26–62 mos	S, C, A
		22 MR	26–62 mos	
Sigman et al.	1986	18 AUT	34–75 mos	S, C
		18 MR[a]		
		18 NOR[a]		
Sigman & Ungerer	1984(a)	14 AUT	$M = 51.9$ mos	S
		14 NOR[a]		
Sigman & Ungerer	1984(b)	16 AUT	39–74 mos	S, A
		16 MR	32–80 mos[a]	
		16 NOR	16–25 mos[a]	
Stone et al.	1990	22 AUT	39–68 mos	S, A
		15 MR	48–72 mos	
		15 HI	36–72 mos	
		19 DLD	36–68 mos	
		20 NOR	36–73 mos	
Tilton & Ottinger	1964	13 AUT	43–79 mos	A
(also Weiner, Ottinger,		12 MR	39–76 mos	
& Tilton, 1969)		18 NOR	43–71 mos	
Wetherby et al.	1989	3 AUT	30–52 mos	S, C
		4 MR	30–35 mos	
		4 DLD	19–29 mos	
Studies Employing Parental Report				
DeMyer et al.	1967	30 AUT	2–7 yrs	S, A
		30 NOR		
Ohta et al.	1987	141 AUT	2–12 yrs[b]	S, C, A
		33 MR	1–12 yrs	
Stone & Lemanek	1990	20 AUT	39–68 mos	S, A
		14 MR	48–72 mos	
Volkmar et al.	1986	50 AUT	28 mos–33 yrs[b]	S, C, A
Wing	1969	27 AUT	5–15 yrs[b]	S, C, A
		15 MR	4–15 yrs	
		11 DLD-R	8–15 yrs	
		10 DLD-E	7–16 yrs	
		15 BL/DF	4–14 yrs	
		25 NOR	4–15 yrs	

[a]Mental age match.
[b]Retrospective parent report.
AUT = Autistic, SCZ = Childhood schizophrenic, MR = Mentally retarded, NOR = Normal,
APDD = Atypical pervasive developmental disorder, DLD = Developmental language disorder
(E = Expressive, R = Receptive), HI = Hearing impaired, BL/DF = Blind/Deaf.
S = Social, C = Communication, A = Activities/Interests.

autistic children than for mentally retarded, language-disordered, or sensory-impaired (i.e., blind or deaf) children (Ohta, Nagai, Hara, & Sasaki, 1987; Wing, 1969). Cross-sectional data obtained by Ohta et al. (1987) suggest that social relating problems are most common in autistic children between the ages of 4 and 9 years. These authors found that the percentage of parents reporting problems with interpersonal relationships was 22% for 2 to 3 year olds, 60% for 4 to 6 year olds, 58% for 6 to 9 year olds, and 35% for 10 to 12 year olds. Based on these results, one might surmise that social relating problems first become salient to the majority of parents during the mid-to-late preschool years. It is possible that early social relating behaviors of autistic children are not characteristically impaired (or at least are not *perceived* as impaired by parents). Further support for this supposition is provided by Stone and Lemanek (1990), who found no differences between autistic children and mentally retarded children in parental reports of early relating behaviors, such as responding to praise and attention and participating in simple social games, such as pat-a-cake or peek-a-boo.

Eye contact is a social behavior that has been the object of much interest. In the Volkmar et al. (1986) study, the majority of parents of young autistic children (94%) reported that their children avoid eye contact. However, results of a recent experimental investigation by Mundy and colleagues suggest that eye-to-eye gaze in autistic children varies with the situation and may at times occur *more* frequently in these children (Mundy, Sigman, Ungerer, & Sherman, 1986). This study reported that autistic children demonstrated more eye contact toward quiet, inactive adults and toward adults following a tickle game, compared with mentally retarded and nonhandicapped children; in contrast, they showed less frequent use of eye contact to initiate joint attention with adults, i.e., sharing attention while holding a toy or while watching an active mechanical toy.

Other aspects of joint attention, such as pointing to and showing objects, are also exhibited less frequently by autistic children than by developmentally matched peers. These deficiencies have been observed during interactions with experimenters as well as caregivers, and have led several authors to propose that a deficit in the development of joint attention, or indicating skills represents a significant feature of autistic children at the preschool age (Mundy et al., 1986; Sigman, Mundy, Sherman, & Ungerer, 1986; Wetherby, Yonclas, & Bryan, 1989).

The manner in which autistic children receive and display affection also differs from that of nonhandicapped children. Volkmar and colleagues (1986) found that the majority of parents described their young autistic children as emotionally distant (92%). Most parents also reported that their children fail to show affection or interest in being held (78%), or that they ignore (64%) or withdraw from (54%) affectionate overtures. However, other responses to affection often attributed to autistic children, such as becoming limp or rigid when held, were endorsed by less than half of the parents questioned (36% and 43%, respectively). Interestingly, many autistic children do demonstrate appropriate responses to affection; 56% of parents reported responsive smiling and 54% reported that their autistic children cuddle when held (Volkmar *et al.*, 1986).

Information regarding the attachment behavior of young autistic children is available from parental reports as well as from observational studies. The majority of parents report that their autistic children seem not to need their mothers (68%) and are unaware of their mother's absence (58%) (Volkmar *et al.*, 1986). However, recent attachment studies have concluded that these children do show evidence of attachment to their mothers in experimental situations; that is, they exhibit different behaviors with their mothers versus strangers, and they show increased approach behavior upon reunion with their mothers. Results regarding the presence of distress behavior upon separation, however, are less conclusive (Shapiro, Sherman, Calamari, & Koch, 1987; Sigman & Ungerer, 1984a). A relationship between attachment behavior and symbolic play skills has been found for autistic children, suggesting that more advanced levels of symbolic abilities may be required in order for autistic children to develop attachment behavior (Sigman & Ungerer, 1984a).

Peer Relationships

Deficient relationships with peers have also been described for this age group. Parental reports indicate that more autistic children than mentally retarded children demonstrate poor relationships in peer group situations (Ohta *et al.*, 1987). Peer problems appear to increase in prevalence during the preschool years; Ohta *et al.* (1987) reported that the percentages of parents reporting peer problems at ages 2 to 3, 4 to 6, 6 to 9, and 10 to 12 were 17%, 40%, 44%, and 10%, respectively.

Differences between autistic and mentally retarded children have been found for several specific peer behaviors: watching other children, imitating the movements of other children at play, playing cooperatively with another child, playing simple group games, joining in play with other children, and following rules in simple games (Stone & Lemanek, 1990). Fewer reciprocal peer interactions relative to mentally retarded children also have been observed clinically (Sherman, Shapiro, & Glassman, 1983).

Imitation Behavior

Imitation has been referred to as a basic cognitive deficit specific to autism (Prior, 1979). Empirical investigations of the imitative abilities of young autistic children have explored body imitation (e.g., imitating movements such as touching one's nose), vocal imitation (e.g., repeating sounds or words), and motor imitation (e.g., imitating the use of objects). In all areas, the performance of autistic children has been shown to be weaker than that of other groups of handicapped and nonhandicapped children (DeMyer *et al.,* 1972; Sigman & Ungerer, 1984b; Stone *et al.,* 1990). Moreover, autistic children's performance on motor imitation tasks is inferior to their performance on other sensorimotor tasks (e.g., object permanence) (Dawson & Adams, 1984). Among autistic children, body imitation seems to be more difficult than motor imitation (DeMyer et al., 1972), and better imitators tend to be more socially related and more likely to have language skills (Dawson & Adams, 1984).

The importance of motor imitation skills in differentiating young autistic children from others was demonstrated by Stone *et al.* (1990). In a discriminant analysis between an autistic group and a group consisting of mentally retarded, hearing impaired, and language impaired peers, imitation behavior alone was found to account for 70% of the variance in group membership. Parental report of motor imitation behaviors also has revealed differences between autistic children and mentally retarded peers (Stone & Lemanek, 1990).

Although deficiencies in imitation skills seem to characterize young autistic children, there is evidence that these skills improve with age (Garfin, McCallon, & Cox, 1988). Consequently, deficient imitation may be more evident during the preschool years than during later stages of development.

Communication

Although numerous deficits in communicative functioning have been reported for autistic children, little research has focused on children at the preschool level. Much of our knowledge in this area derives from parental reports. Since this topic is covered in more detail elsewhere in this volume (see Chapter 5), this section will provide only a brief overview of communication in preschoolers.

Delayed speech and/or other speech problems are the most common early symptoms of autism (Ohta et al., 1987). These symptoms are reported more frequently by parents of autistic children (84%) than by parents of mentally retarded children (61%) (Ohta et al., 1987). Wing (1969) found that difficulties in the comprehension of speech were more common in autistic children relative to mentally retarded, expressive language disordered, and normal children; however, no differences between autistic children and receptive language disordered or sensory-impaired children were obtained. The majority of parents of autistic children in Volkmar et al.'s (1986) study reported that their children demonstrated the following speech characteristics: poor speech tone or rhythm (71%), pronoun confusion (66%), repeating questions instead of answering them (60%), repeating words or phrases out of context (66%), and asking for things by repeating sentences or questions (55%). Only 30% of the parents reported that their autistic children consistently used words, phrases, or sentences to communicate (Volkmar et al., 1986).

Direct observations of autistic children have revealed differences from other groups in their functional use of communication, i.e., the purposes of communication and the forms that communication takes. Communication samples have revealed that young autistic children communicate less often for the purpose of establishing joint attention than language impaired, mentally retarded, and normal children (Wetherby et al., 1989). Moreover, autistic children are less likely to use pointing or eye contact to request out-of-reach toys and less likely to give objects to their caregivers to request help, relative to mentally retarded and normal peers (Mundy et al., 1986; Sigman et al., 1986).

Restricted Activities and Interests

This is a broad category that includes many different types of behaviors: play and use of objects, insistence on sameness and routines, stereotyped body movements, and unusual sensory interests. With the exception of the first area, most of our information is derived from studies employing parent report methodology.

Play/Use of Objects

The preschool autistic child's play skills and use of objects have received considerable research attention. Experimental studies have revealed that young autistic children demonstrate less appropriate, less diverse, and more repetitive play than mentally retarded children or normal children (Sherman et al., 1983; Stone et al., 1990; Tilton & Ottinger, 1964). They engage in more oral manipulation and less combinational use of toys (Tilton & Ottinger, 1964). Studies investigating developmental levels of play have found that autistic children demonstrate functional play less often than mentally retarded, language impaired, hearing impaired, or nonhandicapped preschoolers (Mundy et al., 1986; Sigman & Ungerer, 1984b; Stone et al., 1990). More frequent use of functional play is associated with better language skills in autistic children (Sigman & Ungerer, 1984b).

Conclusions regarding symbolic play are less clear. Investigators have generally failed to find differences in symbolic play between autistic children and their nonhandicapped peers in free play settings, although less frequent use of symbolic play relative to mentally retarded and normal children has been observed in more structured situations (Mundy et al., 1986; Sherman et al., 1983; Sigman & Ungerer, 1984b; Stone et al., 1990). However, some authors have noted that low levels of symbolic play are exhibited by all groups of children in experimental situations (Mundy et al., 1986; Stone et al., 1990). Accordingly, deficiencies in functional play may be more meaningful than deficiencies in symbolic play in observational studies of preschool-aged autistic children.

Parental reports of their children's play skills are generally consistent with the results of experimental investigations. Autistic children demonstrate less variety in their play, and more perseverative, nonconstructive play (e.g., spinning or mouthing objects) than normal children (DeMyer, Mann, Tilton, & Loew, 1967). Wing (1969) found that a lack of appropriate play was reported more commonly for autistic children than for mentally retarded, language disordered, and normal children; however, no differences from sensory impaired children were found. Similarly, DeMyer *et al.* (1967) found that parents of autistic children reported significantly less appropriate play with toys than normal children. However, appropriate play with various toys was reported for roughly half of the children in the autistic sample. The one exception occurred with regard to doll play; only 10% of autistic children (contrasted with 76% of the normal children) reportedly demonstrate appropriate play with dolls.

Volkmar *et al.* (1986) found that the proportion of autistic children reported to demonstrate a normal interest in toys was low (22%). Parents in this study reported a number of deviant behaviors related to play and the use of objects: ignoring toys (92%), bizarre use of toys (73%), repeated rearranging or ordering of toys (57%), attachments to unusual objects (72%), and preoccupation with spinning objects (75%). The percentages of children reported to demonstrate perseverative behaviors in the DeMyer *et al.* (1967) study were somewhat lower, ranging from 20% to 50% for different behaviors.

With respect to symbolic or pretend play, fewer parents of autistic children (35%) report their children to engage in make-believe activities compared with parents of mentally retarded children (86%) (Stone & Lemanek, 1990). Dramatic play with dolls and dramatic role-playing activities are also reported substantially less frequently for autistic children than for normal children (3% vs. 67% and 30% vs. 90%, respectively) (DeMyer *et al.*, 1967). DeMyer *et al.* (1967) compared maternal report information with direct observations for 10 play behaviors, and obtained an average of 72% agreement (range = 29%–100%) between the two methods.

Sensory Abnormalities

Three types of sensory abnormalities in autistic children have been described: hyporeactivity, heightened awareness, and heightened sensitivity to sensory stimulation (Ornitz, Guthrie, & Farley, 1978). Information gathered from parent reports reveals that disturbances of each type occur frequently in autistic samples. Volkmar *et al.* (1986) found that large proportions of young autistic children were described as hypo-reactive to auditory and pain stimulation; 81% reportedly demonstrated a lack of responsiveness to sounds and 56% were minimally respon-sive to pain. Heightened awareness to visual and tactile sensations were also reported: the majority of autistic children were overly preoccu-pied with minor details of objects (67%), with watching their hands and fingers (62%), and by staring into space (54%), and 56% showed an unusual interest in textures. Heightened sensitivity to auditory stim-ulation (i.e., becoming disturbed by loud noises) was also reported by 53% of the parents surveyed. Wing (1969) found that sensory ab-normalities in vision and proximal senses (i.e., touch, pain, taste, and smell) were reportedly more common for autistic children than for mentally retarded, language disordered, or normal children, but no dif-ferences between autistic children and sensory impaired children were found. Abnormal responsiveness to sounds also failed to differenti-ate the autistic from the receptive language impaired or sensory im-paired children.

Motor Stereotypies

Overactivity and restlessness are reported commonly by parents of young autistic children; rates as high as 85% were found in the Volkmar *et al.* (1986) study. Ohta and colleagues (1987) reported that hyperactivity represented one of the most common early symptoms of autism as well as mental retardation, although the rate was almost twice as high for autistic children. The same authors also found that hyperactivity in autistic children appears to decrease with age; the lowest rates (25%) were reported by parents of 10- to 12-year-old autistic children.

The most common motor stereotypes described by parents of young autistic children are: arm, hand, or finger flapping (52%), rock-ing one's body or head (47%–65%), toe-walking (43–57%), and twirl-ing or whirling (37%–50%) (DeMyer *et al.*, 1967; Volkmar *et al.*, 1986). Wing (1969) found that abnormal body movements occurred more commonly in autistic children relative to all of her comparison groups except the sensory impaired children.

Insistence on Sameness

Very little empirical information is available regarding behaviors indicative of a need for sameness or routine. However, Wing (1969) found that attachment to objects and routines differentiated young autistic children from all other comparison groups. Volkmar *et al.* (1986) found that the most frequently endorsed behavior within this category was becoming disturbed or upset by new, unfamiliar places; this behavior was reported by 62% of parents of autistic children. Less than one-half of the parents questioned reported their children to become upset by strangers (36%) or by environmental changes (48%). Ohta *et al.* (1987) found no differences between autistic children and mentally retarded children in the presence of unusual habits or patterns. However, cross-sectional data suggest that these behaviors may become more apparent with increasing age. The percentages of parents reporting this symptom for children between 2 to 3 years, 4 to 6 years, 6 to 9 years, and 10 to 12 years were 8%, 35%, 36%, and 45%, respectively.

CONCEPTS AND STRATEGIES OF ASSESSMENT

In the assessment process, consideration needs to be given to sources of information, areas to evaluate, and strategies and techniques. It is also helpful to consider how assessment of the preschooler differs from the older autistic child.

How Assessment Differs from the Older Child

In many respects, assessment approaches for young children should be similar to those used for the older child. The major areas of communication, social development, cognitive development, and motor skills should be assessed (Watson & Marcus, 1988) and the normal developmental perspective understood and taken into account. There is perhaps greater emphasis on examining play and imitation skills than with elementary age children and certainly adolescents or adults. Comparisons with what is normally expected at a particular age are more important than when the child is older and useful skill function assumes greater primacy. Although structure and behavior management are essential to obtain a good performance with the preschooler, there is also a need to allow opportunities to observe natural play and social responsiveness. The young autistic child is less familiar with routines and basic rules, has a shorter attention span, and is more easily upset by separation. With lower functioning young children, there may be fewer clear passes on the developmental test and the examiner may leave the testing room with mainly observations and partially completed tasks as the only data from which to draw conclusions. The examiner, then, often has to rely on clinical judgment as much as formal test results with this age group. The assessment situation, therefore, requires even greater ingenuity, flexibility, and adjustment than with the older child.

With respect to assessment instruments, language-based tests are even less appropriate than with the older child for whom their utility has often been questioned (Marcus & Baker, 1986). Infant development measures such as the Bayley Scales (Bayley, 1969) are used more frequently with the preschooler whose skills often fall well within the normative range of this test. At TEACCH, for individualized assessment the Psychoeducational Profile Revised (PEP-R) (Schopler, Reichler, Bashford, Lansing, & Marcus, 1990) provides diagnostic, developmental, and educational information for youngsters whose functioning may be as low as 6 to 9 months and as high as 6 years. With its downward extension into the early preschool years the PEP-R enables the examiner to systematically evaluate beginning imitation, language, and cognitive skills, fundamental areas of development whose delays and deviances are central to an understanding of the young child with autism. At the same time, the PEP-R has a section on assessing atypical behaviors associated with autism, including relating and affect, use of materials, sensory deficits, and unusual use of language and communication. Combining the data from the developmental and behavioral components results in a comprehensive overview of the child's similarities to and differences from the normal child of his or her age. Thus, the use of the PEP-R helps further the understanding of the nature of autistic behavior and functioning in the very early years.

Sources of Information

There are basically three sources of information in the assessment process: direct testing using scales such as the PEP-R or Bayley Scales (see Watson and Marcus, 1988 for a summary of various test instruments), report from home or school which should include a measure of adaptive functioning such as the Vineland Adaptive Behavior Scales (Sparrow, Balla, & Cicchetti, 1984), and observations in a natural setting such as the home, school, or day-care setting. Behavior observation scales designed for use with autistic children (e.g., Krug, Arick, & Almond, 1979; Schopler, Reichler, & Renner, 1986) can be helpful in organizing information obtained in this way. Parents should be considered the primary source with the young child, both in terms of current functioning and early development. Parents have the daily appreciation for the subtle problems that may not appear in a formal examination. If they have other children, parents have a normative perspective that may be lacking in the one-to-one with an adult. In addition, the findings and conclusions from the evaluation have to relate to the parental concerns and match their perceptions, even if their understanding and interpretation differ from the professional's. For example, on a clinic imitation task the child very likely would fail to copy an action on demand, but at home might demonstrate deferred imitation such as pushing a vacuum cleaner. A comprehensive assessment integrates these various sources of data, clarifying possible discrepancies and raising issues to be explored over time in the context of an appropriate treatment program.

Management Strategies and Techniques

In the direct assessment of the young autistic child, both flexibility and attention to behavioral management methods are required. The nature of the child's communication, social, and attentional and organizational deficits make it necessary for the examiner to be ready to adjust and adapt testing techniques to obtain an optimum performance. In addition, a well-managed assessment session enables the examiner to gather a wide range of both formal and informal data to provide a complete and clear picture of the child. Problems in assessment and methods of dealing with them have been described elsewhere (Lansing, 1989; Marcus & Baker, 1986; Marcus, Lansing, & Schopler, in press) and will only be briefly discussed in this chapter. Problems that interfere with the assessment process include the child's inconsistencies in motivation and understanding of contingencies; deficits in sensory processing, organization and attention; unevenness of developmental functioning; and lack of understanding of basic social rules and means of communication. These problems tend to be more acute for preschoolers than for older autistic children. What helps in reducing some of the effects of these disruptive behaviors and learning deficiencies is providing a consistent structure that facilitates the child's understanding of what is expected. This includes the use of a clear visual and testing structure, appropriate task sequencing, use of prompts when needed, concrete and meaningful rewards, and communication geared to the child's level with maximum cues. What the examiner learns in the process of adding structure and gaining control over the situation becomes valuable additional information in the formulation of the case.

Normal Developmental Perspective

As noted earlier, keeping a perspective on what is normal for a child at a particular age is helpful in understanding the atypical and irregular development of the child with autism. Watson and Marcus (1988) provided such a comparison in terms of Wing's triad of social, communicative and imaginative functioning (Wing, 1981). Table 7-2 adapts the Watson and Marcus data to illustrate how such a comparison can be made and examined in two ways. First, by looking at a comparison across a time segment, such as language development from 12 to 24 months, the progress of normal development is contrasted with the limited and restricted development of the young autistic child. With normal children a wide range of words and word combinations along with increased number of functions can be observed; by contrast, autistic language development is slower, with inconsistencies and a lack of questions. A second use of this approach is to examine patterns over time to get a sense of the development of the autistic process. For example, the use of imaginative abilities in the autistic child from 8 to 36 months of age can be noted for the failure of symbolic play to develop fully or with elaboration, the continuation of repetitive, perseverative actions and movements, and the discrepancy between certain cognitive or motor skills and creative play with toys.

Implications from Empirical Studies

In attempting to clarify the nature of social development in autism at any given age, two general classes of behaviors acquire prime im-

Table 7-2. Normal and Autistic Development during Preschool Years*

Age (months)	Language and Communication: Normal Children	Language and Communication: Autistic Children	Imaginative Abilities Autistic Children
8			Repetitive motor movements may predominate waking activity
12	First words emerging Use of jargon with sentence-like intonation Language most frequently used for commenting on environment and vocal play Uses gestures plus vocalizations to get attention, show objects, and make requests	First words may appear, but often not used meaningfully Frequent, loud crying; remains difficult to interpret	
18	3- to 50-word vocabulary Beginning to put 2 words together Overextension of word meanings (e.g., "daddy" refers to all men) Uses language to comment, request objects and actions, and get attention Also pulls people to get and direct attention May "echo" or imitate frequently		
24	3 to 5 words combined at times ("telegraphic" speech) Asks simple questions (e.g., Where Daddy? Go bye-bye?)	Fewer than 15 words, usually Words appear, then drop out Gestures do not develop; few point to objects	Little curiosity/exploration of environment Unusual use of toys—spins, flips, lines up objects
36			Mouthing of objects often persists No symbolic play Continuation of repetitive motor movements (rocking, spinning, toewalking, etc.) Visual fascinations with objects—stares at lights, etc. Many show relative strength in visual/motor manipulations, such as puzzles

*Adapted from Watson and Marcus (1988).

portance: inappropriate or unusual behaviors that occur frequently in autistic children and rarely in other groups, and appropriate behaviors that are rarely seen in autistic children but occur commonly in other groups. Few social behaviors of autistic preschoolers can be said to fit into either class, primarily because studies employing adequate comparison groups are lacking. For example, although several unusual relating behaviors are commonly reported in autistic children (e.g., ignoring people, avoiding eye contact, acting emotionally distant), the degree to which they occur in other handicapped groups has not yet been determined. These data are critical for the purpose of differentiating autistic individuals from children who demonstrate overlapping symptomatology (e.g., language impaired children). Moreover, high proportions of autistic children also demonstrate normal relating behaviors, such as cuddling when held. Perhaps the most definitive conclusion that can be drawn at this point is that the time has come to discard traditional notions of pervasive lack of affection and attachment in autistic children. Thus, the observation of behaviors such as clinging to one's mother in the waiting room or becoming upset upon separation should not lead one to rule out a possible diagnosis of autism.

The quality of peer relationships in autistic preschoolers is another area that requires further investigation. In particular, observational studies are lacking. With respect to parent report information, the available literature suggests the superiority of specific, behaviorally-focused questions to more general or global approaches. It is also important to note that many parents may not have adequate opportunities or experience upon which to base judgments regarding peer relationships; consequently, it may prove valuable to obtain supplementary information from day care personnel or preschool teachers.

Two social behaviors do seem to be particularly important in the diagnosis and assessment of young autistic children: joint attention behaviors and imitation skills. Both behaviors have been found to be deficient in autistic children of comparable mental age, and might be easily incorporated into conventional assessment procedures. The child's use of joint attention behaviors might be assessed by parent or teacher report and/or careful behavioral observations during unstructured activities. Specific behaviors to look for would be the child's use of pointing, showing objects, or eye contact to engage the examiner's attention more directly, by integrating a series of motor imitation tasks into the evaluation. Suggestions for specific tasks can be found in DeMyer *et al.* (1972).

Many recent investigators have taken a functional approach to communication assessment; that is, they have looked beyond a child's speech characteristics (e.g., Wetherby *et al.,* 1989). Indeed, a thorough communication assessment should include determination of the child's means of communication (e.g., speech, gestures), the purposes for which he or she communicates (e.g., to request objects, give information), and the contexts in which he or she is most likely to communicate (e.g., during mealtimes, with the teacher) (see Watson, Lord, Schaffer, & Schopler, 1989, for further details regarding communication assessment). Such assessment information can be gathered by conducting parent interviews, by observing children unobtrusively, and/or by setting up structured situations designed to elicit communication (e.g., placing a desired food out of the child's reach; see Wetherby & Prutting, 1984, and Wetherby *et al.,* 1989, for examples of situations).

It is striking that no observational data is available for this age group vis-à-vis many of the behaviors within the category of restricted interests and activities, i.e., sensory abnormalities, motor stereotypies, and insistence on sameness. Such information may be collected relatively easily, through the use of behavioral rating scales, such as the Childhood Autism Rating Scale (CARS) (Schopler *et al.,* 1988). Indeed, such instruments can also provide valuable data regarding changes in autistic symptomatology with age (cf. Garfin *et al.,* 1988). The one characteristic that may be particularly difficult to observe within a clinic setting, however, is the child's need for sameness and routines; such information may therefore be better obtained through parent or teacher reports.

Results regarding play skills suggest that observations during semi-structured play can provide valuable information of potential diagnostic use. In particular, deficient functional play skills may be detected by observing the child's use of toys, such as a play telephone, musical instruments, a comb and brush, building blocks, and toy cars. Dolls and stuffed animals can be used to collect additional information about symbolic play skills (see Sigman & Ungerer, 1984b for details). However, the absence of symbolic play may be of limited diagnostic value in this age group due to its infrequent occurrence in most preschool children in clinical/experimental settings. Information regarding specific symbolic play behaviors may be more reliably obtained through parental report techniques.

The interpretation of information regarding a child's use of toys can be somewhat difficult. Appropriate toy use is seen in many autistic children, whereas rates of inappropriate toy use may be too low to be of clinical use. Thus the reliance on multiple sources of assessment information that cut across diverse areas of functioning is critical to the process of accurate diagnosis and evaluation.

ASSESSMENT AND TREATMENT PLANNING

The ultimate purpose of a comprehensive assessment is to facilitate intervention. With young autistic children, it is essential that the parents not only be directly involved in the assessment process as providers of information, but that they are the first and most important recipients of test results and interpretation (Marcus & Schopler, 1987). As has been repeatedly demonstrated, parents can be effective agents in the treatment and education of their autistic child (Schopler, Mesibov, Shigley, & Bashford, 1984), and this is especially true during the preschool years, when motivation and energy are strong. Intervention begins during the assessment phase when parents should be given candid answers to their questions, including statements about diagnosis. Parents are far less fragile than often assumed by professionals, and frankly and sensitively presented information about their child will enable them to start to take positive steps in helping their child.

Test results should be linked to the specific questions raised by the parents in a preliminary conference or prior written information. Typically, parents are concerned about lack of or limited speech development, behavior problems usually in the form of noncompliance, or any number of developmental lags. Although not always explicitly stated at the outset as a question, parents usually are interested in knowing about diagnosis and, of course, what can be done to help. If the parents have, on the basis of reading or other sources of information, some understanding and awareness of autism, the diagnosis can be given with the developmental and behavioral data to support it. For the majority of parents, however, who are anxious, uncertain, and hopeful, it is better to carefully discuss the individualized assessment data, covering the primary features of autism and then indicate that such a pattern led to this diagnosis. Allowing ample time for further explanation and high-lighting the child's strengths and potential for learning and improve-ment help build a base for the treatment process.

In this initial conference with parents, there are a few points worth emphasizing that have implications for intervention. First, it is impor-tant that parents recognize that their child's language problems encom-pass receptive as well as expressive delays. Parents often are less aware of the centrality of language comprehension or assume that their child understands what they say. The lack of speech is far more obvious than the receptive problems which are often interpreted as misbehavior or poor attention. Secondly, parents need to make the distinction between their child's language and communication problems. As with receptive language, the deficits in all aspects of communication are less apparent or may be attributable to stubbornness or personality traits like "having a one-track mind." A third point of emphasis is the need for parents to take an active, structured teaching approach with their child. A corol-lary of this is that the natural parenting techniques generally effective with normal children are far less useful with the autistic child. Parents have often partially come to this realization by noting that their typical discipline methods have not worked and that it is very difficult to engage their child in normal play and learning situations. A fourth point with the parents of the young preschooler is to balance optimism about the future with the practical reality of the significance of the current pattern of disabilities and need for intervention.

Based on the evaluation, both general and specific treatment goals can be generated. The full assessment should lead to recommendations about the type of school program, specialized help in language and motor development, further evaluation of possible medical factors in-cluding etiological issues, and parent training and counseling. Areas addressed for educational intervention might include language and com-munication, with emphasis on listening attention and receptive under-standing, expressive verbal and nonverbal language, and the use of spontaneous communication at whatever level is currently understood by the child; self-help, leisure play skills, and independence; imitation, cognitive, and preacademic skills; social skills and behaviors; and or-ganized work skills, including attention span, task completion, and the recognition of consequences.

Specific suggestions for programming linked to these broader goals should come directly from an analysis of the test data, both in terms of performance and behavioral observations. The PEP-R (Schopler *et al.*, 1990) has the advantage of integrating these various types of data, including the use of the "emerge" in its scoring system. By looking at the child's overall pattern of successes, failures, and emerging abilities in the context of an understanding of the major deficits of autism, the intervention can be developed from the skills, behaviors and concepts the child already has or has a partial ability to achieve. The assessment information will indicate what is easy for the child, what is slightly new or difficult, and what is clearly above the child's level. Since treatment and education is carried out primarily by parents and teachers, it is important to give recommendations that can be understood clearly, that are specific, and that are practical to carry out in the child's home and school.

CONCLUSION

Careful and thorough assessment of the preschooler with autism is an essential first step in the development and planning of a comprehensive treatment and education program. In this chapter we discussed the importance of establishing a clear diagnosis, communicating results openly with parents, and linking assessment data to intervention methods. The review of the research literature relevant to the major assessment areas illustrated the relationship between clinical and empirical approaches as well as the gaps in our current understanding of autism. Ongoing collaboration between researchers, clinicians, and families in the developmental assessment of the preschool autistic child will continue to provide both challenges and rewards.

REFERENCES

American Psychiatric Association. (1980). *Diagnostic and statistical manual of mental disorders.* (3rd ed.). Washington DC: Author.

American Psychiatric Association. (1987). *Diagnostic and statistical manual of mental disorders* (3rd ed., rev.). Washington, DC: Author.

Bayley, N. (1969). *Bayley scales of infant development.* New York: Psychological Corporation.

Dawson, G., & Adams, A. (1984). Imitation and social responsiveness in autistic children. *Journal of Abnormal Child Psychology, 12,* 209–226.

DeMyer, M. K. (1979). *Parents and children in autism.* New York: John Wiley & Sons.

DeMyer, M. K., Alpern, G. D., Barton, S., DeMyer, W. E., Churchill, D. W., Hingtgen, J. N.,

Bryson, C. Q., Pontius, W., & Kimberlin, C. (1972). Imitation in autistic early schizophrenic and non-psychotic subnormal children. *Journal of Autism and Childhood Schizophrenia, 2*, 264–287.

DeMyer, M. K., Mann, N. A., Tilton, J. R., & Lowe, L. H. (1967). Toy-play behavior and use of body by autistic and normal children as reported by mothers. *Psychological Reports, 21*, 973–981.

Garfin, D. G., McCallon, D., & Cox, R. (1988). Validity and reliability of the Childhood Autism Rating Scale with autistic adolescents. *Journal of Autism and Developmental Disorders, 18*, 367–378.

Kanner, L. (1943). Autistic disturbances of affective contact. *Nervous Child, 2*, 217–250.

Krug, D. A., Arick, J. R., & Almond, P. J. (1979). *Autism screening instrument for educational planning.* Portland, OR: ASIEP Educational Co.

Lansing, M. D. (1989). Educational evaluation. In C. Gillberg (Ed.), *Diagnosis and treatment of autism* (pp. 151–166). New York: Plenum Press.

Marcus, L. M., & Baker, A. F. (1986). Assessment of autistic children. In R. J. Simeonsson (Ed.), *Psychological assessment of special children* (pp. 279–304). Boston: Allyn & Bacon.

Marcus, L. M., Lansing, M. D., & Schopler, E. (in press). Assessment of the autistic and pervasive developmentally disordered child. In D. J. Willis & J. L. Culbertson (Eds.), *Testing young children.* Austin, TX: Pro-Ed.

Marcus, L. M., & Schopler, E. (1987). Working with families: A developmental perspective. In D. Cohen, A. Donnellan, & R. Paul (Eds.), *Handbook of autism and atypical development* (pp. 499–512). New York: Wiley.

Mesibov, G. B. (1983). Current perspectives and issues in autism and adolescence. In E. Schopler & G. B. Mesibov (Eds.), *Autism in adolescents and adults* (pp. 37–53). New York: Plenum Press.

Mundy, P., Sigman, M., Ungerer, J., & Sherman, T. (1986). Defining the social deficits of autism: The contribution of non-verbal communication measures. *Journal of Child Psychology and Psychiatry, 27*, 657–669.

Ohta, M., Nagai, Y., Hara, H., & Sasaki, M. (1987). Parental perception of behavioral symptoms in Japanese autistic children. *Journal of Autism and Developmental Disorders, 17*, 549–563.

Prior, M. R. (1979). Cognitive abilities and disabilities in infantile autism: A review. *Journal of Abnormal Child Psychology, 7*, 357–380.

Rutter, M. (1978). Diagnosis and definition of childhood autism. *Journal of Autism and Developmental Disorders, 8*, 139–161.

Schopler, E. (1983). New developments in the definition and diagnosis of autism. In B. B. Lahey & A. E. Kazdin (Eds.), *Advances in clinical child psychology* (Vol. 6, pp. 93–127). New York: Plenum Press.

Schopler, E. (1987). Specific and nonspecific factors in the effectiveness of a treatment system. *American Psychologist, 42*, 376–383.

Schopler, E., Mesibov, G. B., Shigley, R. H., & Bashford, A. (1984). Helping autistic children through their parents: The TEACCH Model. In E. Schopler & G. B. Mesibov (Eds.), *The effects of autism on the family* (pp. 65–81). New York: Plenum Press.

Schopler, E., Reichler, R. J., Bashford, A., Lansing, M. D., & Marcus, L. M. (1990). *Individualized assessment and treatment for autistic and developmentally disabled children: Vol. 1, Psychoeducational profile revised.* Austin, TX: Pro-Ed.

Schopler, E., Reichler, R. J., & Renner, B. R. (1988). *The childhood autism rating scale.* Los Angeles: Western Psychological Services.

Shapiro, T., Sherman, M., Calamari, G., & Koch, D. (1987). Attachment in autism and other developmental disorders. *Journal of the American Academy of Child and Adolescent Psychiatry, 26*, 480–484.

Sherman, M., Shapiro, T., & Glassman, M. (1983). Play and language in developmentally disordered preschoolers: A new approach to classification. *Journal of the American Academy of Child Psychiatry, 22,* 511–524.

Sigman, M., Mundy, P. Sherman, T., & Ungerer, J. (1986). Social interactions of autistic, mentally retarded, and normal children and their caregivers. *Journal of Child Psychology and Psychiatry, 27,* 647–656.

Sigman, M., & Ungerer, J. A. (1984a). Attachment behaviors in autistic children. *Journal of Autism and Developmental Disorders, 14,* 231–244.

Sigman, M., & Ungerer, J. A. (1984b). Cognitive and language skills in autistic, mentally retarded, and normal children. *Developmental Psychology, 20,* 293–302.

Sparrow, S. S., Balla, D. A., & Cicchetti, D. V. (1984). *Vineland adaptive behavior scales.* Circle Pines, MN: American Guidance Service.

Stone, W. L., & Lemanek, K. L. (1990). Parental report of social behaviors in autistic preschoolers. *Journal of Autism and Developmental Disorders, 20,* 513–522.

Stone, W. L., Lemanek, K. L., Fishel, P. T., Fernandez, M. C., & Altemeier, W. A. (1990). Play and imitation skills in the diagnosis of young autistic children. *Pediatrics, 86,* 267–272.

Tilton, J. R., & Ottinger, D. R. (1964). Comparison of the toy-play behavior of autistic, retarded, and normal children. *Psychological Reports, 15,* 967–975.

Volkmar, F. R., & Cohen, D. J. (1988). Classification and diagnosis of childhood autism. In E. Schopler & G. B. Mesibov (Eds.), *Diagnosis and assessment in autism* (pp. 71–89). New York: Plenum Press.

Volkmar, F. R., Cohen, D. J., & Paul, R. (1986). An evaluation of DSM-III criteria for infantile autism. *Journal of the American Academy of Child Psychiatry, 25,* 190–197.

Watson, L., Lord, C., Schaffer, B., & Schopler, E. (1989). *Teaching spontaneous communication to autistic and developmentally handicapped children.* Austin, TX: Pro-Ed.

Watson, L., & Marcus, L. M. (1988). Diagnosis and assessment of preschool children. In E. Schopler and G. Mesibov (Eds.), *Diagnosis and assessment in autism* (pp. 271–301). New York: Plenum Press.

Weiner, B. J., Ottinger, D. R., & Tilton, J. R. (1969). Comparison of the toy-play behavior of autistic, retarded, and normal children: A reanalysis. *Psychological Reports, 25,* 223–227.

Wetherby, A. M., & Prutting, C. A. (1984). Profiles of communicative and cognitive-social abilities in autistic children. *Journal of Speech and Hearing Research, 27,* 364–377.

Wetherby, A. M., Yonclas, D. G., & Bryan, A. A. (1989). Communicative profiles of preschool children with handicaps: Implications for early identification. *Journal of Speech and Hearing Disorders, 54,* 148–158.

Wing, L. (1969). The handicaps of autistic children: A comparative study. *Journal of Child Psychology and Psychiatry, 10,* 1–40.

Wing, L. (1981). Language, social, and cognitive impairments in autism and severe mental retardation. *Journal of Autism and Developmental Disorders, 11,* 31–44.

Wing, L. (1988). The continuum of autistic characteristics. In E. Schopler & G. B. Mesibov (Eds.), *Diagnosis and assessment in autism* (pp. 91–110). New York: Plenum Press.

8

Medical Syndromes in Young Autistic Children

LAWRENCE T. TAFT

INTRODUCTION

Autism is a syndrome that is behaviorally defined. These characteristic symptoms may be manifestations of a specific disease that results in dysfunctions of the central nervous system. When a physician identifies an infant or young child as being autistic, he or she attempts to define an etiology.

Autism is due to an organic dysfunction of the central nervous system (Ritvo & Freeman, 1984). We subclassify the organic etiologies into "idiopathic" and known causes. The latter designation implies the knowledge of a specific structural or biochemical abnormality of the brain that can be proven. Many of these will be discussed in this article. The diagnosis of an idiopathic disorder is made only when the known causes are excluded. What is required for the designation of "unknown etiology" is the absence of high-risk factors that cause brain damage, a negative neurological exam, and appropriate neuroinvestigative studies. Many cases of autism classified as "idiopathic" may prove to be secondary to genetic influences.

This article will restrict itself to a review of developmental disor-

LAWRENCE T. TAFT • Division of Developmental Disabilities, University of Medicine and Dentistry of New Jersey, Robert Wood Johnson Medical School, New Brunswick, New Jersey 08903.

Preschool Issues in Autism, edited by Eric Schopler *et al.* Plenum Press, New York, 1993.

ders of the central nervous system that have often been associated with autism. These include phenylketonuria, congenital rubella, tuberous sclerosis, Fragile X syndrome, Rett syndrome, posthypsarrhythmia, cerebral lipidosis, and the Lesch–Nyhan syndrome and account for 15 to 20 percent of individuals with the diagnosis of Autism.

PHENYLKETONURIA

Phenylketonuria (PKU) is a disorder of the metabolism of the essential amino acid phenylalanine (Jervis, 1954). It occurs in 1 out of 14,000 pregnancies and is transmitted as a somatic recessive trait. If the parents are carriers, one out of four children, whether male or female, will have the disorder. Fortunately, the disorder can now be treated successfully if recognized in early infancy. Each of the 50 states mandate testing of newborns to identify infants with the problem. Consequently, the classical clinical picture of an untreated phenylketonuric child is uncommon. Anecdotally, approximately 20 years ago, I saw many early recognized children with PKU who were placed on a low phenylalanine diet in infancy. I observed in my office that they were hyperactive and impulsive but did not show evidence of classical autistic behavior. When I visited Israel, where PKU is very rare among Ashkenazi Jews, but relatively common in Yemenite Jews, I had the opportunity to visit a Yemenite village that had a few children with PKU who were being treated with a phenylalanine-free diet. Unfortunately, these cases had been recognized very late and the children were intellectually impaired. I saw three children from different families and each one of these handsome Yemenite children was quite aloof, avoided direct eye contact, had no expressive language, and did not use gestures to make his/her needs known. They were relatively quiet in contrast to the hyperactive children I had seen in the United States. I initially interpreted this quiet, but socially isolated behavior of the Yemenite PKU children to be secondary to the child-rearing practices of the Yemenite families. In fact, I tried to make some inquiries as to the practices of the Yemenites to determine any differences from traditional middle-class, American child rearing practices. When I returned home and made an effort to observe a few untreated PKU children, autistic behaviors were quite evident. Thus, the early treatment most likely not only prevented intellectual deterioration but the development of autistic behaviors (Levy, 1986). One could be suspicious that a child may have phenylketonuria if the skin and hair color is lighter than the parents'. Also, children with untreated phenylketonuria will frequently have a musty smell to the skin and to the urine. There is a simple urine test to screen for this metabolic disorder.

INFANTILE SPASMS: HYPSARRHYTHMIA

Over 20 years ago there was a report of four children who had infantile spasms and abnormal electroencephalograms (EEG), classified as hypsarrhythmia. These children, at 1 and 2 years of age, showed classical symptoms of infantile autism (Taft & Cohen, 1971).

An infantile spasm is a type of seizure that may occur in infants from a few months to 19 months of age. It mimics colic in the sense that the baby will suddenly double up in a flexor posture and may let out a scream. These spasms are instantaneous, although they may be repeated in series. Not infrequently, the same spasm may be the extensor type in which the trunk will stiffen in extension. The brain wave is frequently abnormal and, when it is to a degree that the background rhythm between the seizure discharges is abnormal, the pattern is called "hypsarrhythmia" (a Greek word meaning mountainous arrhythmia).

There are many causes of infantile spasms. Frequently it is due to previous brain injury, such as the case of a baby with a static encephalopathy secondary to a birth injury. In about one third of cases, the spasms begin in an infant who, prior to onset, was developing normally; in the first week or so after the onset the neurodevelopmental exam is normal and neuroinvestigative studies do not elucidate the cause. The so-called idiopathic infantile spasms frequently will cease spontaneously at age 3 to 4, but the children will manifest persistent mental retardation. A small percentage of these children will manifest a classical picture of infantile autism. Of four of the children in the initial report, two had movies taken of them prior to the onset of the seizures. The infants appeared to be sociable and normally adaptive. When the seizures started they regressed developmentally and, after the seizures stopped, they showed autistic behaviors. Of concern was that the autism may have been secondary to the adrenocorticotrophic hormone (ACTH) treatment given for the seizures. ACTH increases the production of cortisone, which has been known to cause psychotic behavior. The knowledge that the other two patients did not receive ACTH, but still developed infantile autism tended to rule out the possibility that the autism may have been secondary to an iatrogenic cause. It is now the consensus that the cerebral dysfunction associated with infantile spasms may have a role in the development of the autistic syndrome.

TUBEROUS SCLEROSIS

Tuberous sclerosis (TS) is one of the neurocutaneous syndromes in which abnormalities of the nervous system and the skin coexist. The skin and nervous system are both derived from the primordial tissue ectoderm, which may explain the concomitant pathologies of these two tissues. TS is a genetic disorder with dominant transmission, usually with incomplete expressivity. The clinical picture and course of TS vary greatly. Infants will often present with infantile spasms as described in the section above. The clue that the TS may be present is the finding of vitiligo spots, which are the areas of depigmentation of the skin, usually a few millimeters in size and often ash-leaf in shape. The other way one becomes suspicious of this disorder is the knowledge that the mother or the father or a sibling has signs of the disease.

There are four major ways that TS may be manifested: mental retardation, cutaneous lesions, seizures, and tumors of the brain and other organs. The characteristic skin lesions, adenoma sebacceum, are not seen until after 1 year of age. They are usually easily recognized by 5 years of age. The lesions are angiofibromas that occur over the butterfly area of the face and over the chin. Another, less common type of skin lesion are small fibromas that are seen under the skin and have a propensity for occurring around the nail beds (periungual region), on the gingiva, and over the trunk. A solitary lesion called a shagreen patch is also diagnostic of TS. It is a slightly elevated, irregular, verrucous, grayish-brown patch measuring 1 or 2 cm, and is situated in the midline over the lumbosacral area. The tumors of the intracranial type are giant cell astrocytomas, which occur around the ventricles and protrude into them. They are usually multiple and do not cause increased intracranial pressure. They may be calcified and the calcifications can be seen on the CT scan, even in children 1 year of age. Other types of tumors occur in the retina, skin, lungs, kidneys, and bones. In regard to the bone, there is a diagnostic cysticlike lesion in the bones of the phalanges of the hands that become manifest around puberty.

Children with TS may manifest autistic behaviors (Lawlor & Maurer,

1987). This is seen more commonly in those children whose initial presenting symptom was infantile spasms. The clue that an autistic child may have TS is by observation of the characteristic skin lesions. The knowledge that the youngster had a seizure disorder in infancy is also helpful.

The exact neuropathological insult causing the autistic syndrome is unknown. Nonspecific treatment can prevent the progression of the disorder.

FRAGILE X SYNDROME

Lubs (1969) reported on a family of three generations with four retarded males. He had noted that, on the X chromosome of each of these males, there appeared to be a very small satellite attached by a thin thread to the end of the long arm. Not all the X chromosomes had this abnormality, but up to 50% did. The abnormal morphologies could only be observed if the cells were grown in folic acid-deficient culture media (Hageman, Smith, & Mariner, 1983).

It is believed that in 5% to 10% of autistic males, Fragile X is found. Recently Fragile X has been reported in females. The characteristic clinical finding in males with Fragile X is markedly enlarged testes. Stigmata which, in many cases, give a characteristic facial appearance to Fragile X males, are macrognathia, macrootia (large ears), a long face, and high arched palate. However, like the enlarged testes, these facial characteristics may not be evident until after puberty (Churdley & Hageman, 1987).

Fragile X syndrome is not always associated with autism or retardation. It has also been identified in children with mild learning disabilities. Fragile X is not transmitted in a classical sex-linked recessive genetic pattern, but rather modified genes may play a role in the phenotypic expression of autism.

RETT SYNDROME

Over 25 years ago Rett (1966) described two girls who were autistic, but showed some unusual stereotyped hand movements and later in life developed a progressive neurological disorder. Hagberg,

Aicardi, Dias, and Ramos (1983) expanded on the knowledge of this syndrome by reviewing 35 cases (Table 8-1).

The course of the disease has been divided into a number of stages (Hagberg & Witt-Engerstrom, 1986). The disease is limited to girls. The onset usually occurs between ½ to 1½ years of age. A female infant will be developing normally until there appears to be a slowing and almost an arrest in development. There will be a decrease in attempts to communicate through gestures or words and a gradual loss of eye contact. It will become evident that the circumference of the head, which had been growing normally, has decelerated. Stereotypic hand-waving movements may appear. In Stage II, from 1½ years to 4 years of age, there is marked regression, with more prominent and characteristic patterns developing. The children appear to manifest autistic behaviors with lack of eye contact. This is accompanied by severe dementia. The abnormal hand movements usually are seen. There may be a tendency to constantly hold the hands clapped and move them as if washing or twirl the hands beside the head. Stereotyped patterns in the use of the hands such as pulling the hair, or tapping the chin or other parts of the body may be present. The children will not use their hands for normal play or daily living activities. This lack of hand use has been ascribed to an apraxic difficulty. Many of the children have episodic hyperventilation and facial grimacing. Seizures will have their onset during this stage, and may be of the myoclonic type. Naidau *et al.* have described the youngsters as having visual, tactile, and auditory agnosia. During Stage III, the preschool to early school years, the autistic behaviors diminish, but gross motor dysfunction becomes evi-

---

Table 8-1. Classical Rett Syndrome: Diagnostic Criteria for Inclusion

1. Female sex
2. A normal pre- and perinatal period; essentially normal psychomotor development through the first 6, and often 12 to 18 months of life
3. Normal head circumference at birth
   Deceleration of head growth (and thus, of brain growth) between age ½ to 4 years
4. Early behavioral, social and psychomotor regression (loss of achieved abilities); evolving communication dysfunction and dementia
5. Loss of acquired purposeful hand skill through ages 1 through 4
6. Hand wringing-clapping-'washing hand' stereotypies appearing between ages 1 through 4
7. Appearance of gait apraxia and truncal apraxia/ataxia from ages 1 through 4
8. Diagnosis tentative until age 3 to 5 years

dent. This takes the form of gait apraxia or a truncal ataxia. Also at this stage, the epileptic symptoms become more prominent. Scoliosis has been noted in Stage IV, which Hagberg calls a late motor deterioration stage, noted between 5 and 25 years. The youngsters become wheel-chair-bound due to the motor handicap, and spasticity appears. The adolescent with Rett syndrome will be noted to stare and have an "unfathomable gaze."

It has been thought that the sporadic appearance of Rett syndrome may indicate a dominant mutation with the abnormality on the X chromosome (which is lethal in the hemizygote state). However, two similarly affected sisters with the same mother have been reported (Hagberg & Witt-Engerstrom, 1986).

There is no marker for Rett syndrome. Biochemical studies of cerebral spinal fluid (CSF), blood, urine, and tissue cultures have been unrevealing. Computer tomography (CT) scans and magnetic resonance images (NMR) are usually within normal limits. Evoked responses and nerve conductions have been normal. Tissue from brain biopsies have not revealed pathologies or biochemical abnormalities. Initially, serum ammonia elevations were reported, but there has been no recent confirmation of this.

A girl with autistic symptoms who shows any of the following should be closely assessed for the possibility of Rett syndrome: (a) decelerated growth of the head; (b) social, language, and motor regression; (c) loss of purposeful hand skill; (d) hand wringing-clapping-washing stereotypies; and (e) gait apraxia and truncal ataxia.

LESCH–NYHAN SYNDROME

This group of children appear normal at birth, but during the second half of the first year of life, they show a delay in psychomotor development and retardation becomes apparent. Approximately one year later extrapyramidal symptoms of the dystonic-athetoid type become manifest. During the first 2 to 3 years of life, those with the disorder lose interest in their surroundings, develop poor eye contact and do not use verbal language as a method for communication and social interaction. Often these children are diagnosed as autistic because they demonstrate many symptoms of this progressive developmental disorder.

The main clinical symptom that makes one suspect Lesch–Nyhan syndrome is involuntary self-injurious behavior, usually restricted to biting fingers, arms, and lips (Lesch & Nyhan, 1964). The author has personally noted that these youngsters often beg for help to keep from compulsively biting themselves.

Within the next 5 to 10 years the children develop a progressive neuromuscular disorder with the onset of spasticity.

The marker for Lesch–Nyhan syndrome is an elevated serum uric acid level. This disorder is considered to be an inborn error of metabolism, with the enzyme deficit being hypoxanthinequanine phosphoribosyl transferase.

The excess uric acid does not seem to be the toxic metabolite. The latter is still unknown. Because of the elevated uric acid, renal calculi and gout are often associated problems. Treatment with allopurinol has a positive effect on the renal calculi and on the symptoms of gait, but no ameliorating effect on the central nervous system symptoms.

INFANTILE NEURONAL CEROID LIPOFUSCINOSIS

This is another neurodegenerative disorder in which infants are normal until 6 to 9 months of age and then gradually show cognitive deterioration. These infants develop seizures and visual failure secondary to pigmentary deterioration of the retina. They also have a delay in the growth of the head and become microcephalic. Intellectual deterioration and visual handicap initially may cause a clinical presentation that fits into the autistic spectrum (Allen, Dyken, Berg, Lochman, & Swaiman, 1982).

Helpful in making this diagnosis is the knowledge that there is a progressive degenerative disease, abnormalities of the electroretinogram, and visual evoked responses. Between 2 to 4 years of age evidence of a progressive central nervous system disease emerges when an ataxic gait, poor vision, and retinal pigmentation are manifested.

The diagnosis can be made by using the electron microscope to identify "fingerprint bodies" as inclusions in lymphocytes. On skin biopsy, curvilinear storage material is seen beset in histiocytes.

Prognosis is extremely poor. Most children continue to regress in motor skills and, after a few years, are in a vegetative state intellectually.

SUMMARY

This review describes a few of the medical conditions that may be associated with the autistic syndrome. Further studies hopefully will lead to the teasing out of other causes. In addition, we must identify the structural or biochemical abnormality common to all the causes that is the "final common pathway" leading to the autistic syndrome.

REFERENCES

Allen, R. J., Dyken, R. R., Berg, B. O., Lochman, L.A., & Swaiman, K. F. (1982). Degenerative disorders of the central nervous system. In K. F. Swaiman & F. S. Wright (Eds.), *The practice of pediatric neurology* (p. 910). St. Louis: Mosby.

Chen, S. (1987). Autism in children with congential rubella. *Journal of Autism and Childhood Schizophrenia, 1,* 33–47.

Churdley, A. E., & Hageman, R. J. (1987). Fragile X syndrome. *Journal of Pediatrics, 10,* 821–830.

Hagberg, B., Aicardi, J., Dias, K., & Ramos, O. (1983). A progressive syndrome of autism, dementia, ataxia, and loss of purposeful hand use in girls: Rett's syndrome report of 35 cases. *Annals of Neurology, 14,* 471–479.

Hagberg, B., & Witt-Engerstrom, I. (1986). Rett syndrome: A suggested staging system for describing impairment profile with increasing age towards adolescence. *American Journal of Human Genetics, Supplement, 1,* 47–59.

Hageman, R. J., Smith, A.C.M., & Mariner, R. (1983). Clinical features of the Fragile X syndrome. In R. J. Hageman & P. M. McBogg (Eds.), *The Fragile X syndrome: Diagnosis, biochemistry and intervention* (pp. 17–53). Dillon, CO: Spectra.

Jervis, G. A. (1954). Phenylpyruvic oligophrenia. In D. Hooker & C. C. Hare (Eds.), *Genetics and the inheritance of integrated neurological and psychiatric patterns.* Baltimore: Williams & Wilkins.

Lawlor, B. A., & Maurer, R. G. (1987). Tuberous sclerosis and the autistic syndrome. *British Journal of Psychiatry, 150,* 396–397.

Lesch, M., & Nyhan, W. L. (1964). A familial disorder of uric acid metabolism and central nervous system functions. *American Journal of Medicine, 36,* 561–570.

Levy, H. L. (1986). Phenylketonuria. *Pediatric Rev., 7,* 269.

Lubs, H. A. (1969). A marker X chromosome. *American Journal of Human Genetics, 21,* 231–144.

Rett, A. (1966). Ube ein eigenastiges eimatrophisides syndrome bei hyperammonamie im kindesalter. *Wien Med Wochenscher, 116,* 723–738.

Ritvo, E. R., & Freeman, B. J. (1984). A medical model of autism: Etiology, pathology, and treatment. *Pediatric Annals, 13,* 293–305.

Taft, L. T., & Cohen, H. G. (1971). Hypsarrythmia and infantile autism: A clinical report. *Journal of Autism and Childhood Schizophrenia, 1,* 327–336.

Taft, L., & Goldfarb, W. (1964). Prenatal and perinatal factors in childhood schizophrenia. *Developmental Medicine and Child Neurology, 6,* 32.

9

Interpreting Results to Parents of Preschool Children

VICTORIA SHEA

INTRODUCTION

The interpretive session in which parents are told the results of their child's developmental testing is the culmination of a complex process of testing, interviewing, analysis of findings, formulation of a diagnostic impression, and generation of recommendations. The session can be a therapeutic turning point for parents, as they are helped to understand their child's needs and plan for his or her future treatment and well-being. Or the session can be a brief, confusing, emotionally devastating lecture about the child's deficits, defects, and labels. The difference derives largely from the professional's commitment to the importance of the interpretive session, and skill in presenting findings in a way that is most helpful to families. The purpose of this chapter is to outline a general approach to interpreting the results of a diagnostic evaluation for mental retardation, autism, and other developmental disabilities (Shea, 1984), and to discuss issues that apply specifically to families of preschool children.

Parents and professionals sit down for an interpretive session about a preschool child's developmental disability in many different settings,

VICTORIA SHEA • Department of Psychiatry, University of North Carolina at Chapel Hill, Chapel Hill, North Carolina 27599-7180.

Preschool Issues in Autism, edited by Eric Schopler *et al.* Plenum Press, New York, 1993.

and their discussions rest on a foundation that varies from family to family. Perhaps the family had been sent for testing by a professional who suspected a developmental problem, but did not inform the family of these suspicions; thus, parents may have been vaguely alarmed, but not fully informed about the nature of the testing or the possible findings. Perhaps the child's testing was part of a routine screening program, which identified previously unnoticed delays or difficulties. Or perhaps parents have been concerned about the child for months or years, so they anticipate that the diagnostic test results may confirm their suspicions and fears.

While some parents of preschool children, particularly those with significant handicaps, fit the latter pattern, to many more parents the diagnosis of a developmental handicap comes as a shock, for several reasons. Parents of young children have a comparatively small number of observations from which to develop concerns about the child's skills. Further, if the child is the parents' firstborn, they may have limited knowledge of normal development with which to contrast this child's skills. In addition, many parents have limited expectations for babies and young children, so that delays in self-care skills, language, or motor development may not be noticed or interpreted as signs of a problem. Thus, parents of young children may approach an interpretive session unprepared to learn of the extent of the child's developmental problems.

Information about the parents' current understanding, questions about the child, prior contact with professionals, and expectations of the interpretive session should be gathered and considered by the professionals before they prepare to present test results and recommendations. Families can easily provide such information, if they are asked. For example: "Did Dr. Smith explain why she thought you should bring Edward to our clinic?" "What was it about Elizabeth that made you think she might need to be tested for a developmental problem? When did you first notice this?" "We would like to talk to you about the results of the pre-kindergarten screening test that Justin took. Had you been concerned about his readiness for kindergarten?"

GOALS AND CONTENT OF THE INTERPRETIVE SESSION

The interpretive session has three goals: (1) to convey information; (2) to assist parents with their emotional reactions to news of their child's handicaps or special needs; (3) to make plans related to the next steps in providing for the child's needs. Thus, there are cognitive, emotional, and behavioral components to a complete interpretive session. Unfortunately, many professionals' training does not prepare them for all of these components. Some professionals overlook parents' emotional needs, which causes families unnecessary pain and a sense of isolation. In other diagnostic settings, emotions and psychodynamics may be overemphasized, while specific information given to parents is minimal. In still other settings, while test results and emotional support are provided, little information is available about practical treatments or resources for additional information. Professionals must strive for all three goals in order for interpretive sessions to be most useful to families.

Physical Setting

The physical setting of the interpretive session is important in creating an atmosphere in which these goals can be met. Professionals should arrange for a private room with comfortable chairs placed so that all participants can see and hear each other. Prior to the interpretive session, professionals should also place a box of facial tissues in the room. Then if the need arises, the professional can hand the box or a tissue to a crying parent, while saying, in effect, "Many parents cry when given this type of bad news. You do not need to be embarrassed about crying. We expect some parents to cry, and are prepared for it."

Content

Parents have a right to know what professionals think about their child. Specifically, parents deserve to know the *names* (labels, diagnoses) of disorder(s) that professionals use in describing their child. The diagnostic terms should be used (and spelled if necessary) at least once with parents. In addition to the name(s) of the disorder(s), parents have a right to understand the *nature* of the problem(s). Thus, the disorder(s) should be explained in language that the parents can understand (for example, "mental retardation means that he is slow in learning and that he is not going to catch up completely to other children his age."). Further, parents should be told how *mild* or *severe* their child's case is.

All professionals know that the skills of children with developmental handicaps can range from borderline normal to profoundly affected; parents, however, may not understand this from hearing the diagnosis alone. Does cerebral palsy mean the child is non-ambulatory? Does mental retardation mean he or she will be unable to work? Does autism mean slightly eccentric?

Past and Future

In addition to name, nature, and severity of the present diagnosis, parents deserve to be given information about both the past and the future. That is, professionals should explain what they know and do not know about the *cause* of the handicap and what they can reasonably expect about its *future course*. In discussing causes, professionals should explore the ideas and fears of the parents related to causation, since these may be idiosyncratic. For example, families may relate emotional stress, physical illness, religious beliefs, or superstitions to the child's problems in ways that might not occur to scientifically-trained professionals. Did the father's depression cause the child's loss of skills? Was the accidental pregnancy responsible for developmental delays? Should the mother not have ridden past a cemetery while pregnant? Should the parents have bought the toddler more toys?

In terms of future course, professionals should help parents begin to anticipate the future, which they may not be able to imagine or may see as bleaker or more hopeful than do the professionals. Some statements about the future can generally be made with relative assurance, and including them in the interpretive session(s) is important to keep the family focused on doing whatever they can to facilitate growth and development. Examples of future topics to consider including in an interpretive session are: Will the child walk? Talk? (if not already doing so). Are there schools for the child? Will the child continue to learn? Can the child be cured? Is this a life-threatening condition?

With preschool children, describing what might be expected in the future is more difficult than with older children. The effects of central nervous system maturation, therapeutic interventions, psychosocial stimulation, love, faith, and luck will continue to influence each child's development uniquely. Therefore, information should be presented in terms of likely outcomes, rather than firm predictions. For example, "Most children who are mildly mentally retarded are able to learn basic academic skills like reading and simple arithmetic." "Children with autism are usually mentally retarded to some degree, and have additional problems with communication and behavior, so they generally need a supervised living situation throughout their life." "Johnny's rate or speed of development has been slow until now, so it's likely that he will continue to develop more slowly than average."

Follow-Up

Family members will think of additional questions or worries after the interpretive session, so professionals should make available to families some mechanism for asking their follow-up questions. This may be a second session, a telephone call initiated by the professional, or encouragement to the family to call the professional if they have questions. In addition, the written report on the child's evaluation could be sent to the family, along with a cover letter that touches on points of confusion or disagreement in the oral interpretive session. For example, "I know you had read somewhere that autism is an emotional disturbance. As we explained to you, the old theory, from forty years ago, was that parents were to blame for their child's autistic behavior, but professionals now recognize that this is not true. Autism is a developmental problem that is caused by the child's brain, not by anything done to him by parents or other caretakers." Another example would be, "We know that some of Billy's scores seemed low to you, and that you were not sure that we had gotten a true picture of his skills. But at least we were able to agree that another year of kindergarten would be the best thing for him, with retesting in the spring before deciding about placement for the following fall."

PRINCIPLES FOR PROFESSIONAL CONDUCT

The content of the interpretive session should be complemented by professional behavior that conveys respect for parents' ideas and sensitivity to their feelings.

Prior Relationship with Parents

Professionals conducting interpretive sessions should have at least some relationship with the parents. Ideally, the parents should have observed the professionals working with their child, and have some confidence that the professionals understand and like their child, and have a good picture of the child's skills and behavior. This ideal scenario is not always possible in clinics, schools, and screening programs where several professionals have worked with the child and family over a short period of time. At a minimum, however, parents should be introduced to all professionals in the interpretive session, and have a few moments to exchange pleasantries and background information before the formal session begins. It is unacceptable for information about the child to be provided by professionals who are essentially strangers to the parents.

Answering Difficult Questions

Professionals should feel comfortable saying, "I don't know," or "I'm not sure." Parents will understand that not all professionals are familiar with their child's condition, that some conditions are rare or unique, and that some questions do not have simple answers. It is far better for professionals to acknowledge their areas of limitation or uncertainty, then help parents find additional information, than to evade questions or give answers that are untrue or of which they are unsure.

Communicating Respect

Respect for the child's and family's individuality should be conveyed to the family throughout the interpretive session. This child is different from any other child the professional has seen. The fact that he or she shares characteristics with other children may be helpful for anticipating the most usual developmental course, but this child has unique physical, psychological, socioeconomic, and family influences. The child's name should be used frequently, and reference made to his age when appropriate (for example, "Since Ryan is almost four and most of his skills are like an 18-month-old . . . ").

Responding to Hope and Denial

Hope—parental optimism which exceeds that of the professionals—is rarely harmful. Professionals should give parents their most honest and complete assessment of the child's needs, problems, strengths, and potential. Parents may or may not believe all the professional says, especially at first. Professionals should not attempt to convince parents of the validity of their ideas. First, they might be wrong. Second, most people need time to adjust in their own way to painful news; this process cannot be rushed by outside forces, particularly intellectual arguments. If the problem is real, almost all parents will grow in their understanding of the problem, as they see additional evidence of it, and as they adjust psychologically to its implications for their lives and their child's life. Third, parental hope and optimism may be beneficial for the child if it results in seeking services, following advice, overcoming discouragement, and generating ideas for helping the child. Certainly, hope can be carried to the extreme of having unrealistic expectations that create additional problems, such as low self-esteem, fear of failure, tantrums, or power struggles. Denial can be taken to the extreme of neglecting treatment and refusing to seek services. If these problems develop, they must be addressed by professionals at a later date. But initial optimism should be presumed to be constructive until it has been proven otherwise.

General Principles

The most important guideposts for professionals in deciding how to present information and respond to questions are honesty and compassion. Many parents (Turnbull & Turnbull, 1985) have written with bitterness about professionals who at first kept information from the parents, only to disclose it later in a cold, abrupt fashion. Similarly, in a survey of 190 parents, Quine and Pahl (1986) found that "parents want to be told as early as possible that there is a cause for concern about their child even though doctors may be unsure of the exact nature of the child's impairment. Parents of children with nonspecific handicaps are particularly vulnerable in this regard" (p. 57). Parents in this survey also complained when they were told in an unsympathetic fashion. Some professionals assume that parents resent all professionals who diagnose developmental disabilities, a hypothesis explored by Cunningham, Morgan, and McGucken (1984) in a paper entitled "Down's Syndrome: Is dissatisfaction with disclosure of diagnosis inevitable?" This study compared parents in two control groups with parents who were first informed of their child's handicaps by professionals following a program of procedures such as a private interpretive session soon after birth, and access to practical information and advice about caring for the infant. Results demonstrated that the answer to the question in the paper's title is "no." Anger and dissatisfaction with the interpretive conference were not inevitable parts of the diagnostic process. Parents in this study were angry about situations and behavior that deserved anger, but when professionals were sympathetic, honest, and helpful, parents expressed complete satisfaction with the interpretive process.

Professionals may have difficulty presenting interpretive information because they are uncertain about how to handle parents' emotional reactions. Parents may become sad, defensive, withdrawn, irritated, or overwhelmed by the diagnostic information, particularly when it comes as a shock. These reactions are normal, and should not be stifled or ignored by the professional. As described in an earlier paper (Shea, 1984) professionals should be prepared to sit quietly and give the parents time to experience their feelings, and should encourage parents to express and discuss their feelings openly. Professionals who have difficulty with expressions of strong emotions within an interpretive session may benefit from discussing their reactions with others who conduct such sessions, or with a personal counselor. If their discomfort cannot be resolved, they should not conduct interpretive sessions, because it is not fair to give families the impression that their feelings are unacceptable, or that they must protect the professional from their honest reactions.

In situations in which a parent's coping skills are limited, it may be useful to have a mental health professional involved in planning and conducting the interpretive session. There may also be circumstances in which a parent's mental or physical health is so precarious that professionals appropriately decide to dilute or withhold interpretive information. However, in most cases withholding information to "protect" parents is patronizing, unnecessary, and occasionally harmful. When professionals themselves confront difficult medical or psychological situations in their own families, they almost always seek out as much information, advice, and support as possible; why should clients deserve any less?

SPECIAL ISSUES IN INTERPRETIVE SESSIONS ABOUT PRESCHOOL CHILDREN

Screening Tests and Preliminary Results

Some interpretive sessions with parents of preschool children will occur in the context of screening programs, in which large numbers of children are tested to identify those at risk for developmental delays or other handicapping conditions. Screening assessments are typically brief, with those children whose scores are marginal referred for more precise and individualized assessment. Such screening programs should have a well thought-out protocol for informing parents of results and providing information about recommended next steps. Otherwise, factors such as impersonal delivery of test results, long delays between screening and further evaluation, limited resources for treatment, false reassurances, or overly sensitive tests (yielding false positive results which later turn out to be benign) may occur and contribute to family turmoil and distress.

However, if parents want to be informed about conditions that professionals suspect before the professionals are certain, then situations will inevitably arise in which the professionals' suspicions do not come to pass. Professionals should present screening results and initial suspicions with the same honesty and compassion that they would with a definitive diagnosis. They should describe the assessment procedures and their thoughts about the child's skills and behavior, identifying clearly their level of certainty in describing findings and explaining the various outcomes that are likely. For example, "Jason's language skills on that test (previously named) were generally around the two year level, and since he is over three, we are concerned that he may have a problem in his understanding and use of language. But it was difficult to be sure, because he didn't want to sit at the table and work on the tests. He pushed the toys away several times, and he often shook his head or turned around when we asked him questions. It is possible that when his behavior is under better control and he is more able to work on the tests, he will score in the average range. But it is also possible that he has a mild developmental problem in language in addition to his behavior problem. So first we need to work on his behavior, then we'll want to retest him."

Most parents can handle being told about suspected problems at least as well as they can handle diagnoses, perhaps because with the former there is the hope that the suspected problem may not in fact exist. In fact, according to many parents who have written about their experiences, the more likely scenario is that the parents attempt to convince the professional (especially the pediatrician) of the validity of suspected developmental problems, rather than the other way around!

Statements about the Future

Many professionals are hesitant to make statements about later functioning based on developmental tests in young children. One reason is the understandable reluctance of professionals to present bad news to families. Causing distress and pain to parents is an uncomfortable task for people in the "helping" professions. Therefore, professionals may look, consciously or unconsciously, for reasons to discount test results that suggest developmental handicaps. A second reason is the fact that tests of normally developing babies and young children are well known not to be good predictors of later academic talents (Sattler, 1988). Early walkers are not necessarily early readers; early talkers do not necessarily enter law school, etc. Combining these two factors may lure some professionals into assuming that early test results are extremely unreliable, and that therefore no statements about future development can or should be made.

This position is being challenged by the growing literature on the correlation of developmental tests of young handicapped children with tests results in later years. Correlations between early and later tests are generally moderate to strong when the early tests are below average (MacPhee, 1982). For example, Maristo and German (1986), following a large group of developmentally delayed infants (average age 11 months) over a year, found correlations on most developmental measures in the range of .74–.93. More than three years later, the correlations between initial evaluation and follow-up were in the range of

.65–.70 for motor and cognitive measures, although the very early language measure was less predictive of later language testing (perhaps because a different measure was used in follow-up testing). In addition to finding that low scores in an area of development were correlated with later low scores in that same area, Maristo and German also suggested that results on developmental tests were so redundant that unless the child had a handicap in a particular motor or sensory area, "it may be assumed that a child will score in the same general range on [all] the different norm-referenced measures" (p. 330). In other words, most delays are global and stable.

Even with children whose development is uneven, it may be possible to anticipate their later development status to some degree. Field (1987) conducted an interesting study of the predictive power of the Leiter International Performance Scale, an old test still used for language-impaired and autistic youngsters. She looked at a sample of children (mean age 4 years, range 37–64 months) whose Leiter scores were significantly higher than their Stanford–Binet IQ's (103 vs. 68). Both measures were correlated with later (mean age 64 months) WPPSI IQ's, but the Leiter overestimated WPPSI scores, while the Stanford–Binet underestimated them. Thus, while early language delays may have masked other cognitive skills on the Stanford–Binet that were picked up on the Leiter, in many cases the Stanford–Binet scores were good indicators of later difficulties. Interestingly, Field suggested that the best predictor of later WPPSI IQ was the average of the Leiter IQ and the Stanford–Binet IQ.

The correlation of early and later developmental test results should not be confused with the ability of early tests to describe a child's overall outcome. Many other factors in addition to level and rate of skill development influence children's eventual developmental status; these include the pattern of strengths and weaknesses, therapeutic interventions, opportunities and experiences, and other indefinable and inestimable qualities that contribute to the uniqueness of each individual and each family. Developmental test scores do not measure factors such as social charm, a sense of humor, resilience in the face of hardship, or courage. Further, developmental tests of young children cannot accurately indicate whether a child will master specific academic, vocational, or self-care tasks. Thus, while we may be fairly sure that a young child with a severe developmental delay will need supervision and special services throughout his lifetime, it would be unreasonable to attempt to anticipate whether or not he would be able, as a young adult, to read the sports page, earn minimum wage, make friends, or prepare a meal.

Inconclusive or Questionable Test Results

Circumstances that bring into question the validity of test scores include sensory or motor limitations, severe non-compliance or inattention during testing, significant discrepancies among tests, scores that are inconsistent with behavioral observations in other settings, or a history of abuse, neglect, or prolonged environmental deprivation (including hospitalization). When such factors are involved, conclusions from a single assessment must be considered to have questionable predictive validity, although they may represent a valid estimate of the child's current skills.

If developmental test scores indicate significant delay, but the clinician does not believe the scores are an accurate reflection of the child's potential, how should the information be presented? Using the guideline of honesty with the parent, the professional can explain what the results were, in what ways they seem valid, in what ways they may not be valid, what recommendations can be made based on the child's current needs, and when retesting might be expected to be more valid and useful. Professionals need to guard against being overly optimistic (e.g., "these results are meaningless and your child will certainly score better next time"), but should equally be on guard against relying on test results with obvious limitations.

Grandparents

Parents of young children are often young themselves, and likely to have strong ties with their own parents and parents-in-law. These grandparents may thus play a significant role in the parents' ideas, feelings, and actions regarding the child's developmental problems. It is not uncommon during an interpretive session for parents to wonder aloud how they will explain the diagnostic information to the grandparents, and what their reactions will be. Parents' distress may increase as they think about the sorrow the news will cause the grandparents.

Alternatively, parents may anticipate that the grandparents will not understand or agree with the findings, will criticize the parents for having the child evaluated, will attribute the child's behavior to poor parenting, or will reject the child if they are told of the child's problems. While all possible scenarios cannot be anticipated, the main point for professionals to remember is that grandparents' reactions may be a major issue for parents, and particularly those of young children; thus part of the professional's responsibility in an interpretive session may be to help parents express their feelings about and deal with the issue of telling the grandparents.

Additional Children

Parents of preschool children are also more likely than parents of older children to consider having additional children. Prediction of the risk of developmental problems in other family members and additional children depends upon accurate and complete medical diagnosis of the child being assessed. This requires evaluation by a physician knowledgeable about developmental handicaps, perhaps working in conjunction with a professional genetic counselor; other non-medical professionals should not attempt to take on this role. They can, however, encourage and help parents obtain further information if they would like to understand the risk factors involved in future pregnancies. This has always been an issue of interest to young families, but recent advances in knowledge about Fragile X syndrome, suggesting that many cases of mental retardation that were previously considered to be of unknown etiology might have a genetic basis, have made genetic counseling even more important and useful than it was five or ten years ago. With Fragile X and with other chromosomal and genetic disorders, the child's siblings may be at risk for carrying genetic disorders, so that genetic counseling might be appropriate for them as well.

CONCLUSION

While the interpretive session may be difficult for everyone involved, it is a necessary and potentially rewarding facet of the parent's relationship with the child and with the professional community. When conducted well, the interpretive session can convey to the parent that there is help and hope for the child, and that the professionals can also be counted on for support, advice, and honest information about the child. The teamwork between parent and professional that begins in the open exchange of information, ideas, and feelings will serve the parent and child well throughout the child's life.

REFERENCES

Cunningham, C. C., Morgan, P. A., & McGucken, R. B. (1984). Down's syndrome: Is dissatisfaction with disclosure of diagnosis inevitable? *Developmental Medicine and Child Neurology, 26,* 33–39.

Field, M. (1987). Relation of language-delayed preschoolers' Leiter scores to later IQ. *Journal of Clinical Child Psychology, 2,* 111–115.

MacPhee, D. (1982). *Prediction of intellectual outcome in childhood from assessments made during infancy.* Unpublished manuscript. (Available from Department of Human Development and Family Studies. Colorado State University, Ft. Collins, CO 80523).

Maristo, A. A., & German, M. L. (1986). Reliability, predictive validity, and interrelationships of early assessment indices used with developmentally delayed infants and children. *Journal of Clinical Child Psychology, 4,* 327–332.

Quine, L., & Pahl, J. (1986). First diagnosis of severe mental handicap: Characteristic of unsatisfactory encounters between doctors and parents. *Social Science and Medicine, 22,* 53–62.

Sattler, J. M. (1988). *Assessment of children* (3rd ed.). San Diego, CA: Author.

Shea, V. (1984). Explaining mental retardation and autism to parents. In E. Schopler & G. B. Mesibov (Eds.), *The effects of autism on the family* (pp. 265–288). New York: Plenum Press.

Turnbull, H. R., & Turnbull, A. P. (1985). *Parents speak out: Then and now.* Columbus, OH: Charles E. Merrill.

10

Early Intervention for Children with Autism and Related Developmental Disorders

CATHERINE LORD, MARIE M. BRISTOL, and ERIC SCHOPLER

It has long been recognized that the learning and accomplishment of developmental tasks occurs at a particularly rapid rate in children in infancy, preschool, and early school years (Havighurst, 1979). Accordingly, the impetus for early intervention for children with developmental disabilities, such as autism, has recently produced a renewed emphasis on preschool intervention and education. This chapter is based on two decades of experience with our program for the *T*reatment and *E*ducation of *A*utistic and related *C*ommunication handicapped *CH*ildren (TEACCH), the only comprehensive statewide system for the study and education of such children (Schopler, in press, 1989; Schopler, Mesibov, Shigley, & Bashford, 1984; Schopler & Olley, 1982). We view the purpose of early intervention as producing maximum adaptation for each child in collaboration with the child's family. In this chapter, we will discuss general issues in the diagnosis and assessment of preschool children with autism and related disorders, and then

CATHERINE LORD • Department of Psychiatry, University of Chicago, Chicago, Illinois 60637. MARIE M. BRISTOL and ERIC SCHOPLER • Division TEACCH, Department of Psychiatry, University of North Carolina at Chapel Hill, Chapel Hill, North Carolina 27599-7180.

Preschool Issues in Autism, edited by Eric Schopler *et al.* Plenum Press, New York, 1993.

briefly describe approaches to diagnosis and intervention employed at the TEACCH program.

COMPARISON OF ISSUES FOR PRESCHOOL VERSUS OLDER CHILDREN WITH AUTISM

Many of the intervention programs currently employed for autistic children originally arose from theoretical and clinical models developed for children entering school or who were already in school (Donnellan, 1980; Everard, 1976). However, the situation and needs of children, particularly those at ages 2 or 3 who are several years from formal school entry, are often quite different from the 6- and 7-year-olds for whom programs were initially designed. A number of factors present special demands for a program providing assessment and intervention for very young children. These factors range from differences in family situations and skill level of the children to differences in professionals' expectations and knowledge of what and how to teach very young children.

Differences in Diagnosis and Assessment

Parents of 2- and 3-year-olds referred for possible autism are often just beginning to realize that there is something significantly different about their child's development from that of other children. Because most autistic children are not different in obvious, physical ways from other preschool children, this recognition can be difficult for parents. Most parents are not aware of how different their children are socially from other children. This is partly because certain kinds of social interaction and communication are just beginning to develop and partly because parents may automatically compensate for their child's difficult or absent social behavior. For example, when the young child is unusually passive, parents may initiate more interaction, and when the child's communication is unclear, parents may actively interpret their meaning. Given such compensations, parents of autistic children often seem to be able to elicit more "normal" interactions than otherwise possible. In addition, many parents, especially those without other children, are often not cognizant of the range and flexibility of normal social behavior. Because normally developing infants and toddlers are not necessarily consistent in using exactly the same combination of social behaviors across time and situation, many parents attribute their children's deficits to normal inconsistency. There is also evidence that some autistic children actually participate in social interactions (e.g., reciprocal vocalizing) more actively as infants than they do in their second or third year (Eriksson & de Chateau, 1992). Regressions in language have also been well documented (Kurita, 1985). Sudden or gradual loss of a child's first words may leave parents wondering "where their real child has gone."

Parental confusion is exacerbated by the fact there is considerable ambiguity in diagnosis of younger autistic children, particularly those under 3 years of age or those who are very delayed in all skills. Toddlers with autism can usually be distinguished from nonhandicapped children by professionals, but it can be difficult at these very young ages to differentiate the qualitative deficits of autism from the severe developmental delays of mental retardation or related disorders (Dahlgren & Gillberg, 1989; Knobloch & Pasamanick, 1975). Young children diagnosed with autism under age 3 years do not typically meet formal diagnostic criteria for autism such as those of ICD-10 or DSM-III-R (Gillberg et al., 1990).

There are also many different reasons besides autism why young children may not be socially interactive or communicate, particularly in the context of a clinic visit or a one-time assessment. Parents often report that their child behaves differently at home. However, even at home, autistic children do not show the range of social and communication skills typical of normal development (Le Couteur et al., 1989; Volkmar et al., 1987). Parents may not be aware of such norms and instead may focus on the discrepancy between the child's behavior at home and at the clinic.

Autism-specific characteristics such as unusual language and play may not distinguish a young preschool child with autism from other children because several other diagnostic groups (e.g., children with severe mental handicap or language disorder) also show limited amounts of directed communication and play. Many autistic children have also not yet developed the obviously repetitive behaviors that are part of the autism syndrome (Lord, Storoschuk, Rutter, & Pickles, 1992). Thus, professionals are often in the position of asking parents to acknowledge

the possibility of a very severe handicap in their young children because of the absence of normally developing behaviors rather than the
presence of clear, unusual development. This can be difficult for parents to accept.

In the past, several years often elapsed between when parents
first became concerned about their child's development and when a
diagnosis of autism was made (Short & Schopler, 1988). Today, a
parent may only mention a vague concern about lack of language in
their 2-year-old to their pediatrician to find themselves referred for
further assessment. Several weeks later they may be presented with a
diagnosis of autism, a lifelong disorder with a guarded prognosis. It is
not surprising that many families take time to accept such a diagnosis.
Decisions about which social and communication delays constitute autism rather than other disorders cannot be made without careful observation and inquiry, and without familiarity with both autism and
the differential diagnosis. It is important to allocate sufficient time both
for the assessment of young children and for discussion of the diagnosis with the family.

Intellectual and developmental scores, while relatively good predictors of later nonverbal intelligence, do not provide adequate discrimination of degrees of mental retardation in young preschool children
(Lord & Schopler, 1989). It is not possible to predict with much certainty which young autistic children will be mildly versus moderately
retarded (Lord, Schopler, & Revecki, 1982). Preschool children with
autism who speak in spontaneous sentences by age 3 and do well (i.e.,
$IQ > 70$) on nonverbal intelligence tests are likely to continue to score
in the same range on intelligence tests and other measures throughout
the elementary school years. However, finding that a 3-year-old with
autism is *not* verbal or does poorly (i.e., $30 < IQ < 50$) on infant developmental tests does not necessarily mean the child will never speak or
will remain severely mentally handicapped. In one study, 50% of nonverbal, autistic 3-year-olds who scored in the severe range of mental
handicap showed increases of more than *30* points when reassessed 5 to
8 years later (Lord & Schopler, 1989).

Scores on early developmental tests are often determined by children's refusal to attempt scorable tasks in the usual way (e.g., a child
mouths blocks rather than trying to build a tower or shows no interest
in stacking cups). This is in contrast to tests for older children where

parents can observe their child attempt an answer and not be able to get it right. Parents of preschool children are also more likely to indicate that their children have never seen similar objects or been in a similar situation (in a small room with a closed door with a stranger presenting a series of toys that come out of a suitcase) than parents of older children for whom tests are more similar to schoolwork (Watson & Marcus, 1988). Thus, although few autistic children labeled as severely mentally handicapped score in the average range of intelligence years later, the scores of many autistic children during school years will increase significantly.

Differences in Family Situation and Approach

Differences in family situations may have more marked effects for children in the preschool years than later on. A 4-year-old with autism who has been asked to leave day care because he is not toilet trained creates different stress for a working single mother than for a mother who is home with her child during the day. First-time parents often have different anxieties and knowledge about child development than parents who have already lived through the early preschool years with one or more other children (Short & Schopler, 1988). Differences among families in the amount of time available, both to work with professionals and within which to devote undivided attention to their young child, cannot be underestimated. Differences in the amount of support, to mothers particularly, both within and outside of the nuclear family, may also be exacerbated in families with young children (Bristol, 1987). These factors are relevant for older children, but again show less variation among families when school becomes a greater factor and when the probability increases that there are other children and the mother is employed outside the home.

Parents differ in their approaches to a diagnosis of their preschool child. Some parents feel strongly that they would like a label or a "worst case scenario," and then work from this knowledge, allowing for the possibility that goals and plans can be shifted in a positive way if the child makes more progress than expected. Other parents are very uncomfortable with their young child being labeled. These families may proceed more effectively by focusing on specific aspects of their child's development and behavior that will respond to treatment, without giving much attention to (or even accepting) diagnostic categories or long-term prognoses. In one study, parents' acceptance of the long-term implications of their moderate to high-functioning preschool children's autism was better predicted by the age of the child (much greater acceptance when the child was 5 years old than 2 to 3 years old) and to a lesser degree by the length of time since diagnosis, than any characteristic of the child, including severity of mental handicap (Lord, 1983). Some of these differences are surely related to family character-istics and some to the characteristics of the child. Working within the style with which the parents feel comfortable is necessary. It is import-ant that professionals refrain from conveying more certain diagnostic pronouncements than the ambiguities of early diagnosis and measure-ment permit. Focusing on the needs of the child and family at the time of diagnosis is the most important factor in beginning a relationship with a family of a young child.

Differences in the Children

Many autistic children in preschool also differ from older autistic children in that they often lack very basic communication skills. They may not come when they are called, may not recognize their names, may have no idea of the notion of carrying out an activity upon request (including nonverbal requests), and may have no concept of "first you do this, and then this happens." Families often adjust to this lack of comprehension and communication without knowing it, so that the child's difficulties are obscured at home or appear different from those observed during preschool. Parents are usually quite accurate in an-swering questions about their child's behavior in specific situations, (for example, "Could you send him into another room to get something not part of the ongoing activity—such as your purse or a book?") They may also supply accurate information on their child's difficulty answer-ing certain questions, but even when parents describe such difficulties accurately, they do not necessarily interpret this information to mean that their child does not understand them.

Safety becomes an issue as autistic preschool children become able to run, open doors, and climb, but do not come when called, understand "no," or comprehend the possible dangers of busy streets or getting lost. On the other hand, very young autistic children can be carried, cuddled, and cajoled in ways much more difficult with a school-age child and may be much less conspicuous if they have a tantrum or cry than an older child.

A final difference in planning for preschool children versus older children with autism is that curricula are often less well-defined in the early ages. Many formal teaching models for autism began with goals of helping children with academic or prevocational academic tasks. These goals are appropriate for some preschool children, but are often too advanced or move too quickly for very young, low-functioning children with autism (Schopler, Reichler, & Lansing, 1980). Often these goals fail to encompass the range or flexibility seen in normally developing children's play at young ages. On the other hand, this flexibility generally arises from creativity exhibited by children themselves, rather than curricula designed to teach it. Thus, strategies to teach autistic children what they will need for academic and vocational work are more readily available than strategies to teach them what they are lacking as young preschoolers. Structured teaching, so important with older children (Schopler, Mesibov, & Hersey, in press), needs special adaptation at the preschool level (to be discussed below). Behavioral models provide useful starting points for adults establishing control of young children's attention and reducing some interfering behaviors, but often offer relatively limited suggestions for gradual acquisition of developmentally based social or communication skills (Lovaas, 1977). Communication curricula based on psycholinguistic research often begin at a point that far exceeds the capabilities and attention span of autistic youngsters whose present "communication age" may be under 6 months.

Recent approaches that emphasize incidental learning (Koegel, Dyer, & Bell, 1987) and building on the communication skills and interests that the children already have (Watson, Lord, Schaffer, & Schopler, 1989) are beginning to fill this gap. Recent intervention models have used play as an endpoint as well as a medium for the acquisition of other skills (Rogers, Herbison, Lewis, Pantene, & Reis, 1986; Wohlfberg & Schuler, 1992). Knowledge about how and whether to incorporate such models into early intervention programs is still needed. In addition, many young autistic children have marked social difficulties even in interacting with competent adults. The most appropriate ways to facilitate peer interactions are not well understood, although models for early intervention have shown positive effects of integrated social interaction programs (Harris, Handleman, Kristoff, Bass, & Gordon, 1990; Odom, Hoyson, Jamieson, & Strain, 1985).

While there are special aspects of dealing with autistic children during preschool years, there are also similarities across age. There is a continued need to coordinate services from community and education programs with the needs of families. Structure in schedule, physical layout, and behaviors of familiar people also makes a difference to autistic children of all age ranges (Schopler *et al.*, in press; Schopler & Olley, 1982). Clear, definable goals with emphasis on practical functional communication and independent activity at whatever level possible are also important parts of the TEACCH model, regardless of whether the student is learning to drop blocks in a can as an example of a directed visuomotor behavior, bring his or her shoes to mother to indicate a desire to go outside, do third grade math problems, or fill out employment applications.

SPECIAL FACTORS FOR PRESCHOOL CHILDREN WITH AUTISM VERSUS OTHER DISABILITIES

Young children with autism share many of the same needs that children with other disabilities and children without handicaps have. These include the need to learn basic self-help and cognitive skills, the need to acquire behaviors that make it easier to learn in a group, such as sitting for a few minutes and taking turns with other children, and the need to learn to carry out tasks on request. In this context, in group or during one-on-one intervention programs, all young preschool children also share the need for warmth and structure offered by teachers with clear goals and the flexibility to instill a joy of learning in their students.

On the other hand, young children with autism differ from children with other handicaps in a number of ways. The most obvious difference is in level of language. When matched on any measure of nonverbal skills, autistic children, particularly in the preschool years, show markedly lower language comprehension and production than children with other disabilities (Lord, Storoschuk, & Rutter, 1992). Autistic children not only have difficulties understanding language in the absolute (that is, knowing exactly what particular words mean out of context), such as in a test of communication skills, but also show more marked difficulties in understanding language in context and making sense of what is happening around them. Similarly, autistic children often have much less interest in peers and may not have the flexibility (seen in children with other developmental disabilities) necessary to sort out beginning peer relations with children their own age. Along the same lines, young autistic children are less likely to imitate and to initiate and show sustained pretend play than are other children of equivalent developmental levels (Lewis & Boucher, 1988; Rogers & Pennington, 1991; Ungerer & Sigman, 1981). In this way, they often require more structure and goals specified in smaller steps than children without autism.

The situation of parents of autistic children is also often somewhat different than some parents of other children with developmental disabilities. In most cases, autistic children do not come from "high risk" families. While there may be genetic components to autism, they are generally not reflected in behaviors or characteristics of parents such as mental handicap or the socioeconomic factors more frequently seen in parents of children with mild mental handicap without autism (Schopler, Andrews, & Strupp, 1979). In addition, as described earlier, in very young children, autism is often an ambiguous diagnosis. Parents may be involved in early intervention programs before a clear diagnosis is made. Even if professionals are certain of the diagnosis, parents are often not. Parents of autistic children may have greater hopes that their children will grow out of their disorder than parents of children for whom a diagnosis was made at birth or early infancy on the basis of physical characteristics rather than behavior (Lord, 1983; Schopler & Reichler, 1972). Altogether, autism is associated with somewhat different needs for children and families in the preschool years than other diagnoses. In order to help these children approximate their learning potential, it is important that these differences be recognized by service providers.

TEACCH SERVICES FOR PRESCHOOL CHILDREN WITH AUTISM AND RELATED DISORDERS AND THEIR FAMILIES

The TEACCH Model

The TEACCH model and its guiding principles have been described in detail elsewhere (Schopler, 1989; Schopler et al., 1984; Schopler et *al.,* in press). Thus, only the components of the TEACCH model particularly relevant for children under 6 years of age will be discussed here. The developmental approach of TEACCH recognized differences between children and also differences within any particular child in the rate and nature of development across different skill areas. This emphasis is very important in planning services for young children. For example, one 3-year-old child with autism may have expressive and receptive language below that of a 6-month-old, fine motor and visual–spatial skills like that of a 20-month-old, and gross motor skills close to age level. Planning for this child needs to take into account this pattern, as compared to another 3-year-old who might have receptive language at a 2-year-old level, expressive language at an 18-month level, visual–spatial skills at age level, and some mild motor delays. Practical issues such as when and how to start toilet training and how to plan for safety must be based on individual developmental patterns.

A second aspect of the TEACCH model is the importance of the family. While it is clearly recognized that each autistic child has special characteristics, goals for treatment are also seen as including the individual child and other family members. Objectives include not only changing the behavior and skills of the child, but modifying the environment to better suit the child's needs. This perspective arises out of a belief that children are best served within their community and within their own families, and that this is made possible by increasing both the flexibility of the child and aspects of the environment (Schopler, 1989). The role of TEACCH is to support the needs of each family in whatever way makes the most sense for it and the child.

A third assumption underlying the TEACCH model is that there is a direct relationship between assessment and intervention. This link is best seen as carried out by therapists who see themselves as "generalists." Assessment should include not only formal testing, but observation and careful collection of information from parents and teachers. Intervention is based on what the child already can do in daily life situations. Altogether, these assumptions lead to a belief in the importance of individualizing programs for children and their families. There is a strong commitment to drawing from a variety of alternatives to find the right place and the right approach for each child in his or her family at a particular time.

TEACCH Center and Preschool Services

There are six regional TEACCH centers in the State of North Carolina each seeing approximately 45 new preschool children each year and a total of about 650 to 700 preschool children at any given time. In TEACCH affiliated classrooms, there are usually 5 children per teacher and an assistant teacher. There are 14 such preschool classrooms in the state. Other children are in noncategorical preschool programs for handicapped children, in day-care centers, regular preschools, and at home. Referrals are made by parents, physicians, teachers, early intervention workers, speech therapists, and other professionals. When a referral is made, a TEACCH therapist contacts the source of referral and the child's parent to determine its appropriateness. Children for whom there is some suspicion of autistic behaviors or a combination of severe language delay and social impairment not accounted for purely by mental handicap are accepted. About 60% to 75% of the children accepted for assessment are later diagnosed as autistic using standard diagnostic criteria (American Psychiatric Association, 1987; Schopler, Reichler, & Renner, 1988). Once assessed, follow-up is based on need, not diagnosis. Children who are not accepted into the program are referred to other resources. If the child is accepted for a full assessment, the assessment begins with a home visit by a therapist in which a standard diagnostic interview is given to the parents (Le Couteur *et al.,* 1989) or in some clinics, a similar but informal interview is given as part of the clinic assessment. In addition, this visit provides a chance to meet the child and to get a sense of the parents' priorities.

A standard diagnostic assessment day includes a team of three people: a clinical psychologist (the clinical director of the center), and two psychoeducational therapists, one of whom works with the child and one who has already interviewed the parent(s) in their home. The latter therapist continues to serve as parent consultant and follows the family through all further contacts. The child's teachers and other professionals working with the child are invited to a staff meeting before the assessment begins. They then observe the assessment through a one-way mirror. The Psychoeducational Profile Revised (PEP-R; Schopler, Reichler, Bashford, Lansing, & Marcus, 1990) is always given first by a psychoeducational therapist. This instrument establishes developmental levels in seven areas. It also allows the therapist to observe the child during a variety of tasks that vary in structure and social-communicative demands. Each item on the PEP-R is scored as "passed" (according to standard criteria), "emerging" (i.e., the child shows some ability to carry out part of the task or carry out the task in a modified fashion), or "failed;" thus, the PEP-R yields a profile of emerging as well as well-established skills.

During this time, the parents are given the Vineland Adaptive Behavior Scales (Sparrow, Balla, & Cicchetti, 1984), and the parent consultant goes over any new concerns; the parents watch the testing through a one-way mirror or may join the child in the testing room, if necessary. After the Psychoeducational Profile is administered, psychological (nonverbal intelligence, standard intelligence) and language tests are given by the clinical psychologist. If appropriate, a structured observational schedule (Prelinguistic Autism Diagnostic Observation Schedule; DiLavore, Lord, & Rutter, 1992) is administered to the child with the help of a parent. This instrument provides an opportunity to observe specific aspects of the child's social behavior such as joint attention, sharing of affect, and imitation with a stranger and with the parent. Parents are then asked to play with their child with toys they have brought from home, and to engage in language or preschool tasks. This enables staff to observe parent-child interactions and to compare the child's reaction with familiar people to that with strangers. This comparison can offer valuable clues for differences in teaching strategies at home and at school. Next, families are sent to lunch and a second staff meeting, including visiting professionals and teachers, takes place. At the end of the day, results are conveyed to the parents by the clinic staff, followed by a written report. A second brief session is scheduled approximately a month later, after the parents have received the reports, to discuss the results and to provide another opportunity to work with and observe the child.

Parents are offered a number of treatment options and encouraged to maintain some contact with their TEACCH center, even if they are not able to participate in a formal treatment program. A school or home visit is often arranged to provide suggestions for behavior management or programming. Also available to the parents is an "extended diagnostic" period in which parents and child return to the clinic for six to eight 1-hour sessions over the course of several months to work as cotherapists with their child.

During the extended diagnostic period, results of the diagnostic evaluation are converted into structured teaching activities for home use. These are based on the seven areas of function assessed by the PEP-R (Schopler *et al.*, 1990) involving motor control (as with puzzles or crayons), communication with objects or pictures (Schopler, Reichler, & Lansing, 1980; Schopler, Lansing, & Waters, 1983), and activities for promoting spontaneous communication (Watson & Marcus, 1988).

Special emphasis is brought to making this structured teaching interaction enjoyable for both child and parent and having the activities relevant to the child's developmental level. The teaching activities are written out for parents to use in daily sessions lasting from 10 minutes to half an hour. The parent takes the teaching activities developed by the staff and is encouraged to make modifications or add activities as informed by this experience. In their return visits, parents demonstrate their use of the teaching program with staff coaching or demonstration. Parents also demonstrate progress and discoveries they have made with staff support and involvement. Through close collaboration between staff and parent, optimum teaching programs are identified. This extended diagnostic is especially helpful with parents of preschool children. These parents are often still quite overwhelmed or confused by the meaning of their child's behavior, and they are torn between letting the child go his or her own way or attempting counterproductive pressure with social behavior such as toilet training.

These structured sessions in which parents are alone with their child and having a good time may improve parental coping effectiveness (Marcus *et al.*, 1978) and carry over to other situations. This extended diagnostic period also often provides constructive collaboration between parents and teachers of the preschool class. This is facilitated by new teachers' attendance in our summer preschool training. In addition, much of the therapists' time is spent coordinating our findings and suggestions with those of other agencies and therapists, most frequently speech pathologists and early intervention workers. Families are encouraged to have a complete medical work-up for their child if this has not been done. In addition, families are directed to family support groups, both specifically for autism, such as the local chapters of the Autism Society of North Carolina, or groups for all developmental disorders, including programs such as "Parent-to-Parent" organizations run out of local hospitals.

TEACCH-Affiliated Classrooms

The principles guiding the TEACCH programs as a whole (Schopler, in press, 1989; Schopler *et al.*, in press) also apply to our preschool classrooms. First is the objective of maximizing adaptation by teaching new adaptive skills. When this process is blocked by a deficit, we develop environmental modifications to accommodate the deficit. This is best achieved with parent–teacher collaboration, individualized assessment of each child, and in the use of structured teaching and behavior management. Structured teaching provides educational continuity from preschool age to adult years (Schopler *et al.*, in press), and also prevents many behavior problems from developing. When we first showed that autistic children learned better with a structured rather than an unstructured learning situation (Schopler, 1989), we also noted that children at earlier developmental levels needed structure more than children at higher levels of functioning. However, just as the diagnosis of autism is more obscure and requires more special consideration at the preschool age than at later ages, so does the use of structured teaching.

The majority of children with autism and related developmental problems share certain learning problems and strengths. They may be disorganized and have problems with remembering events unrelated to their special interests, although special interests and attention can often be converted to useful skills. They often have more trouble processing information through the auditory modality than they do visually. Structured teaching uses visual processing strengths in the four major components, including physical structure of the room; object, word, or picture schedules for reminding the child when classroom activity takes place; a visual work system for learning various tasks and their sequences; and visual organization of instructional materials.

The emphasis in the preschool class, in addition to clarifying diagnostic ambiguities, is on learning to be a student and developing appropriate social and communicative behaviors. Compared with school-aged children, preschoolers are exposed to a wider range of activities. Due to their shorter attention span, daily schedules involve shorter activities. Children spend more time learning and practicing fine and gross motor skills in small groups. Parents are more often involved in the classroom than they are later on. These factors contribute to the greater emphasis on the physical structure aspect of the curriculum and the layout of the classrooms shown by the example in Figure 10-1.

In this figure, there are clear visible indications of where each activity will occur in order to help the student learn to stay in certain areas without prodding from the teacher. Learning activities for teaching cognitive, fine motor, eye hand integration, and organizational skills occur at the tables. Self help skills such as toileting, eating habits, washing hands, wiping tables, and hanging up coats are taught in the upper left-hand corner in or near the bathroom. Expressive communication, receptive language, and social interaction are formally taught in another marked area, but also occur as part of all other classroom activities. Daily schedules clearly help each child learn directions, and those with better visual processing skills can be helped to anticipate changes in activities through the use of objects, pictures, or words. Examples of such schedules are shown in Figure 10-2. Concrete objects (puzzle pieces and a flashlight) are used to help Danny know what activity is next on his schedule. Rob follows a sequence of pictures which he takes and puts in matching pockets in the appropriate areas of his classroom. Johnny has learned to read and can check off and follow a written schedule.

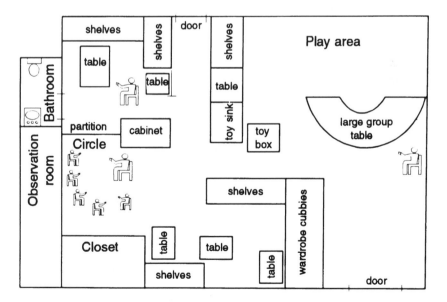

Fig. 10-1. Sample floor plan for preschool demonstration classroom.

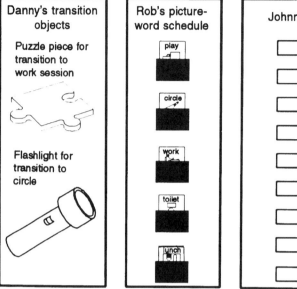
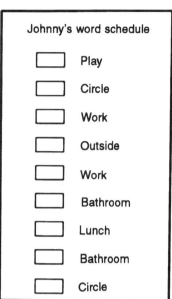

Fig. 10-2. Three types of schedules.

Such activities can be adapted to different levels of communication. They can be used to facilitate transitions from one activity to another. Such schedules are often helpful even for children integrated in the mainstream classroom. Children are also helped to develop independent work behaviors in short, structured work sessions during the school day. Visual work systems (see Figure 10-3) use matching colors, shapes, letters, or numbers to help children know what work is to be done, when they are finished (when the pockets are empty), and what reward they can give themselves when finished (e.g., go to play area). Figure 10-4 shows a picture jig that the child uses to fold pairs of socks, one example of visual organization of materials.

Other classroom facilities are also available. In addition to 14 TEACCH preschool classrooms designed specifically for children with autism or related communication handicaps, there are noncategorical programs for children with disabilities run by school districts and mental health consortiums, and there are integrated programs in which the children with autism participate in regular preschool or day-care centers. Other children are at home with their full-time homemaker mothers

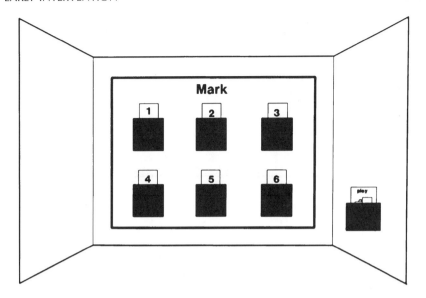

Fig. 10-3. Individual work system.

working with home teaching programs, or are placed in other child-care settings to which TEACCH staff supply consultation as needed.

Parent Involvement

The most intense parent-teacher collaboration occurs when a parent, usually the mother, functions as an assistant teacher in the class-

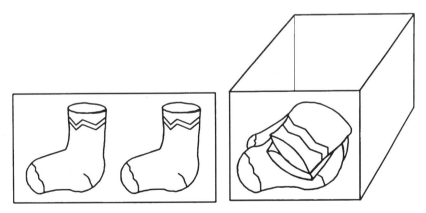

Fig. 10-4. Picture jig.

room once or twice a week. When this parent-teacher collaboration is possible, it can be very helpful for generalizing learning from home to school. Another level of parent involvement consists of classroom observation and participating in home teaching demonstrations. Collaboration is also facilitated by home and school diaries, special birthday celebrations, evening family events, sibling days, field trips, parent-teacher discussions, and ongoing parent support groups.

Structured Teaching and Behavior Management

Structured teaching provides the primary basis for educational continuity in the TEACCH program, as it can be adjusted to individual levels of communication on a continuum from the developmentally impaired to the nonhandicapped. As discussed above, by accommodating the learning environment to the deficits associated with autism, independent functioning of each student is fostered, and many frustrations and behavior problems are avoided. Emphasis is on positive strategies and using structure to minimize difficulties before behavior problems occur. Although the majority of behavior problems are avoided through structured teaching, a combination of cognitive and behavioral interventions are also employed. This strategy of multiple approaches can be illustrated for one of the frequent preschool behavior problems—toilet training. Figure 10-5 presents an illustration using an iceberg metaphor for toileting difficulties.

Above the water line are specific behavior problems such as smearing feces or eliminating in inappropriate places. Below the water line are possible explanatory deficits. By careful observation and parent interviews, an informal assessment is made of antecedent behaviors and circumstances. For example, a child who eliminates in the wrong places may not be recognizing bodily signals in time. If observed holding himself or herself or otherwise indicating awareness of having to go at the same time of day, regular and pleasant trips to the bathroom may be initiated then. If the inappropriate elimination dissipates, the assessment and intervention were correct. If it continues, further observation and interventions are necessary.

Follow-up

Services are available to families at TEACCH from the time of diagnosis through adulthood. Parents of very young children are en-

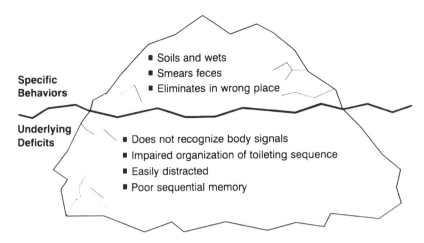

Fig. 10-5. Iceberg metaphor for toileting difficulties.

couraged to seek formal reevaluation at TEACCH or through other resources after a year or two, depending on how rapidly the child is changing and how valid the first assessment was felt to be. After that, follow-up is done on the basis of need. In addition, consultation to other educational and medical programs throughout our cachement area is offered.

SUMMARY AND CONCLUSIONS

In conclusion, three issues can be identified that are central to helping a preschool child with autism through services available through the TEACCH program. First is a reconsideration of the notion of continuum of services. Often programs have been described as providing a continnum of services, meaning that services are available from preschool through adulthood. However, another way of thinking of a continuum of services is to conceive of the continuum as covering a wide range of different approaches and different sites for children within the same age group. Thus, given diverse family situations, differences among autistic children in language level and ability to interact with peers, and differences in what is available in various communities, the TEACCH model supports a continuum of services *within* each age group. Within one community that has good "regular" day care centers, a good medical base, and excellent speech pathologists, TEACCH may be most effective as a backup for early intervention workers who are able to place young autistic children in integrated programs. Children may already be receiving high-quality treatment on a regular basis from private or public health speech pathologists, for whom we can provide consultation or in-service training. In another community, a categorical classroom for autistic children may be developed because of the needs of three or four young children who require high degrees of supervision and intense structure. TEACCH therapists may be actively involved in working with parent volunteers in the classroom. In this situation, the role of TEACCH may be to advocate for reverse mainstreaming and a continued focus on spontaneous communication and social interaction within the specialized setting. In another community, a group of mothers who are at home may each come in biweekly to work as cotherapists with the TEACCH staff; another role of the center may be to provide a mothers' support group as well as a monthly weekend activity group for siblings.

A second, similar point to the idea of a continuum of services within an age group involves coordination with the community. More and more in the last few years, TEACCH therapists have spent substantial amounts of time working with other professionals to develop and implement particular educational plans for individual children and their families. Again, the resources in different communities vary considerably, but in the long run, working with other professionals in the community is more efficient and effective than developing competing programs. Many of the services available in the community, such as early intervention programs, are tied to specific age groups, but have greater resources at any given time than TEACCH does (e.g., the ability to make three home visits a week for several years). It is assumed that the relationship between TEACCH and each family is long-term and not tied to specific services or institutions. For example, over 3,000 people have been served by TEACCH in the last 20 years; a single center may serve over 500 families, about 250 of whom would be actively receiving services. What TEACCH can offer is the continuity of following a child from toddlerhood or early preschool years into school age and adulthood, providing different kinds of service and support as needed.

The third issue is that of theoretical approach and training. While many of the techniques employed in working with young children have arisen out of behavioral traditions, TEACCH continues to emphasize the importance of using these techniques within a developmental frame-work. Structuring the environment using time, space and physical cues is an integral part of the TEACCH model. Readers are referred to other papers describing assessment methods (Marcus & Stone, this volume; Schopler et al., 1990), work with families (Bristol, 1987), and communication curriculum (Watson et al., 1989) for further information. One implication of an eclectic approach is the need for professionals to see themselves to some extent as generalists. While the therapists in TEACCH clinics come from a range of disciplines, including special education, speech pathology, social work, early education, and psychology, they are recruited and hired on the basis of their good social skills with families, interest and ability to work with children, and the ability to think critically and write clearly. In-service and on-the-job training with a variety of autistic children across home, clinic, and school settings provide a base upon which the therapists can build the skills that they acquire with experience.

In conclusion, it has often been easier to describe the deficits of autistic children than it has been to determine the specific aspects of intervention that are effective, particularly over time. It is clear, however, that early social and communication training can improve children's skills, can interrupt and prevent, to some degree, the development of secondary behavior problems, can improve parental skills, and can increase behaviors that children need in order to learn in a school setting (Schopler, 1989). In a variety of ways, young autistic children present a particular challenge in diagnosis and intervention. It is also important to remember that these children are part of families within communities. It is the goal of the TEACCH program to build on the strengths of each child, family, and community to help the child achieve particular goals and to help the family and community cope with the challenge of living with a young child with autism.

REFERENCES

American Psychiatric Association. (1987). *Diagnostic and statistical manual of mental disorders* (3rd ed., rev.). Washington, DC: Author.

Bristol, M. (1987) Mothers of children with autism or communication disorders: Successful adaptation and the ABCX Model. *Journal of Autism and Developmental Disorders, 17,* 469–486.

Dahlgren, S. O., & Gillberg, C. (1989). Symptoms in the first two years of life: A preliminary population study of infantile autism. *European Archives of Psychiatric and Neurological Science, 283,* 169–174.

DiLavore, P., Lord, C., & Rutter, M. (1992). *Prelinguistic Autistic Diagnostic Observation Schedule.* Unpublished manuscript.

Donnellan, A. M. (1980). An educational perspective of autism: Implications for curriculum development and personnel development. In B. Wilcox & A. Thompson (Eds.), *Critical issues in educating autistic children and youth* (pp. 53–88). Silver Springs, MD: US Department of Education.

Eriksson, A., & de Chateau, P. (1992). Brief report: A girl aged two years and seven months with autistic disorder videotaped from birth. *Journal of Autism and Developmental Disorders, 22,* 127–129.

Everard, M. P. (Ed.). (1976). *An approach to teaching autistic children.* Oxford: Pergamon.

Gillberg, C., Ehlers, S., Schaumann, H., Jacobsson, G., Dahlgren, S. O., Lindbloom, R., Bagenholm, A., Tjuus, T., & Blidner, E. (1990). Autism under age 3 years: A clinical study of 28 cases referred for autistic symptoms in infancy. *Journal of Child Psychology and Psychiatry, 31,* 921–934.

Harris, S. L., Handleman, J. S., Kristoff, B., Bass, L., & Gordon, R. (1990). Changes in language development among autistic and peer children in segregated and integrated preschool settings. *Journal of Autism and Developmental Disorders, 20,* 23–31.

Havighurst, R. J. (1979). *Developmental tasks and education* (4th Ed.). New York: Longview.

Knobloch, H., & Pasamanick, B. (1975). Some etiologic and prognostic factors in early infantile autism and psychosis. *Pediatrics, 55,* 182–191.

Koegel, R. L., Dyer, K., & Bell, L. K. (1987). The influence of child-preferred activities on autistic children's social behavior. *Journal of Applied Behavior Analysis, 20,* 243–252.

Kurita, H. (1985). Infantile autism with speech loss before the age of 30 months. *Journal of the American Academy of Child Psychiatry, 24,* 191–196.

Le Couteur, A., Rutter, M., Lord, C., Rios, P., Robertson, S., Holdgrafer, M., & McLennan, J. D. (1989). Autism Diagnostic Interview: A standardized investigator-based instrument. *Journal of Autism and Developmental Disorders, 19,* 363–387.

Lewis, V., & Boucher, V. (1988). Spontaneous, instructed, and elicited play in relatively able autistic children. *British Journal of Developmental Psychology, 6,* 325–339.

Lord, C. (1983, April). *Parents' understanding of the children's development: Observations and expectations.* Paper presented at the biennial meeting of the Society for Research in Child Development, Detroit, MI.

Lord, C., Storoschuk, S., Rutter, M., & Pickles, A. (in press). Using the AD1-R to diagnose autism in preschool children. *Infant Mental Health.*

Lovaas, O. I. (1977). *The autistic child.* New York: Irvington.

Marcus, L. M., Lansing, M. D., Andrews, C. E., & Schopler, E. (1978). Improvement of teaching effectiveness in parents of autistic children. *Journal of the American Academy of Child Psychiatry, 17,* 625–639.

Odom, S. L., Hoyson, M., Jamieson, B., & Strain, P. S. (1985). Increasing handicapped preschoolers' peer social interactions: Cross-setting and component analysis. *Journal of Applied Behavior Analysis, 18,* 3–16.

Rogers, S., Herbison, J., Lewis, C., Pantone, J., & Reis, K. (1986). An approach for enhancing the symbolic, communicative, and interpersonal functioning of young children with autism or severe emotional handicaps. *Journal of the Division of Early Childhood, 10,* 135–148.

Rogers, S. J., & Pennington, B. F. (1991). A theoretical approach to the deficits in infantile autism. *Development and Psychopathology, 3,* 137–162.

Schopler, E. (in press). Behavioral priorities for autism and related developmental disorders. In

E. Schopler & G. Mesibov (Eds.), *Assessment and management of behavior problems in autism*. New York: Plenum Press.

Schopler, E. (1989). Principles for directing both educational treatment and research. In C. Gillberg (Ed.), *Diagnosis and treatment of autism* (pp. 167–183). New York: Plenum Press.

Schopler, E., Andrews, C. E., & Strupp, K. (1979). Do autistic children come from upper middle class parents? *Journal of Autism and Developmental Disorders, 9,* 139–152.

Schopler, E., Lansing, M., & Waters, L. (1983). *Individualized assessment and treatment for autistic and developmentally disabled children: Vol. 3. Teaching activities for autistic children.* Austin, TX: Pro-Ed.

Schopler, E., Mesibov, G., & Hersey, K. (in press). Structured teaching. In E. Schopler & G. Mesibov (Eds.). *Assessment and management of behavior problems in autism.* New York: Plenum Press.

Schopler, E., Mesibov, G., Shigley, R., & Bashford, A. (1984). Helping autistic children through their parents: The TEACCH model. In E. Schopler & G. Mesibov (Eds.), *The effects of autism on the family* (pp. 65–81). New York: Plenum Press.

Schopler, E., & Olley, G. (1982). Comprehensive educational services for autistic children: The TEACCH Model. In C. R. Reynolds & T. R. Gutkin (Eds.), *The handbook of school psychology* (pp. 629–643). New York: Wiley.

Schopler, E., & Reichler, R. J. (1972). How well do parents understand their own psychotic child? *Journal of Autism and Childhood Schizophrenia, 2,* 387–400.

Schopler, E., Reichler, R., Bashford, A., Lansing, M., & Marcus, L. (1990). *Individualized assessment and treatment for autistic and developmentally disabled children: Vol. 1. Psychoeducational profile revised (PEP-R).* Austin, TX: Pro-Ed.

Schopler, E., Reichler, R., & Lansing, M. (1980). *Individualized assessment and treatment for autistic and developmentally disabled children: Vol. 2. Teaching strategies for parents and professionals* (2nd ed.). Austin, TX: Pro-Ed.

Schopler, E., Reichler, R. J., & Renner, B. R. (1988). *The Childhood Autism Rating Scale (CARS),* Los Angeles: Western Psychological Services.

Short, C. B., & Schopler, E. (1988). Factors relating to age of onset in autism. *Journal of Autism and Developmental Disorders, 18,* 207–216.

Sparrow, S., Balla, D., & Cicchetti, D. (1984). *Vineland Adaptive Behavior Scales.* Circle Pines, MN: American Guidance Service.

Ungerer, J. A., & Sigman, M. (1981). Symbolic play and language comprehension in autistic children. *Journal of the American Academy of Child Psychiatry, 20,* 318–337.

Volkmar, F. R., Sparrow, S. S., Gondreau, D., Cicchetti, D. V., Paul, R., & Cohen, D. J. (1987). Social deficits in autism: An operational approach using the Vineland Adaptive Behavior Scales. *Journal of the American Academy of Child and Adolescent Psychiatry, 26,* 156–161.

Watson, L., Lord, C., Schaffer, B., & Schopler, E. (1989). *Teaching spontaneous communication to autistic and developmentally handicapped children.* Austin, TX: Pro-Ed.

Watson, L., & Marcus, L. M. (1988). Diagnosis and assessment of preschool children. In E. Schopler & G. Mesibov (Eds.), *Diagnosis and assessment in autism* (pp. 271–301). New York: Plenum Press.

Wohlfberg, P., & Schuler, A. (1992). *Integrated play groups: Resource manual.* San Francisco: San Francisco State University.

11

Current Practices in Early Intervention for Children with Autism

J. GREGORY OLLEY, FRANK R. ROBBINS, and MARLENE MORELLI-ROBBINS

INTRODUCTION

Over the last 20 years, there has been a veritable explosion in the growth of early intervention programs for young children with handicaps. Starting from a few demonstration programs in the 1960s, to more systematic work in the 1970s, to more data-based replications and encouraging outcomes in the 1980s, we have witnessed a steady increase in the quality and the documented effectiveness of many such programs. This trend has been paralleled by a proliferation of edited books (e.g., Bickman & Weatherford, 1986; Guralnick & Bennett, 1987; Odom & Karnes, 1988), special issues of journals (e.g., Dunst, McWilliam, & Trivette, 1985; Fewell, 1985), and a myriad of reviews on the overall "effectiveness of early intervention" (e.g., Bricker, Bailey, & Bruder, 1984; Bryant & Ramey, 1987; Casto & Mastropieri, 1986; Dunst & Rheingrover, 1981; Farran, 1990; Ferry, 1981; Simeonsson, Cooper, & Schiener, 1982). Reviews have discussed issues pertain-

J. GREGORY OLLEY • Clinical Center for the Study of Development and Learning, University of North Carolina at Chapel Hill, Chapel Hill, North Carolina 27599-7255   FRANK R. ROBBINS and MARLENE MORELLI-ROBBINS • Department of Child and Family Studies, Florida Mental Health Institute, University of South Florida, Tampa, Florida 33612.

Preschool Issues in Autism, edited by Eric Schopler *et al.* Plenum Press, New York, 1993.

ing to the efficacy of early services for children across the diagnostic spectrum, including those with general cognitive delays (Guralnick & Bricker, 1987), Down syndrome (Gibson & Fields, 1984), hearing impairments (Meadow-Orlans, 1987), organic handicaps (Dunst & Rheingrover, 1981), children at risk for developing handicaps (White & Casto, 1984), as well as those with autism (Simeonsson, Olley, & Rosenthal, 1987). The comprehensive review by Simeonsson *et al.* (1987) found that only two programs for children with autism had demonstrated success based on experimentally rigorous designs. These were Strain's LEAP preschool at the University of Pittsburgh (Strain, Jamieson, & Hoyson, 1985) and Lovaas' Young Autism Project at the University of California, Los Angeles (Lovaas, 1987). On the basis of these limited data, the authors tentatively pointed to several components that were associated with effective practices in preschool services for children with autism. These programs were structured, had a behavioral orientation, emphasized parent involvement, began treatment at an early age, provided intensive services, and had a focus on the generalization of newly learned skills (Simeonsson *et al.*, 1987).

Rather than provide another "effectiveness of early intervention" review, this chapter describes 11 contemporary preschool programs and examines their contributions to knowledge and practice in light of current issues. For instance, researchers and practitioners are beginning to ask what specific approach to early intervention is effective for what group (or subgroup) of children. Karnes and Johnson (1988) elaborated on this point and went on to charge researchers with asking: "What intervention options are available, what situations are most conducive to implementing the option, and what resources are needed to implement it adequately?" (p. 288).

The framework for this chapter is based in part on two recent reviews that suggest future directions for early intervention services and research for children with a variety of handicapping conditions. Karnes and Johnson (1988) focused on six themes: (1) social validity—are the changes seen as a result of early intervention truly meaningful? (2) triangulation—the use of multiple measures in evaluating early intervention programs; (3) the need for replication across different subjects, behaviors, and settings; (4) dependent measures—an overreliance on testing, and a singular focus on child data to the exclusion of instruments that gauge the impact of the intervention on the family;

(5) independent variables—the need for better descriptions of our interventions and how they are implemented; and (6) impact—the importance of disseminating results to a wider audience, especially practitioners and policymakers in the field.

A second review by Guralnick (1988) pointed to five related issues: (1) clearly specifying the subject sample and program characteristics; (2) selecting an educational or developmental model that is well matched to the needs of the population; (3) broadening parent involvement beyond the unidimensional role of "parents as teachers" by providing parents with coping strategies and expanding the resources available to them; (4) more closely examining intensity as an important variable related to outcome; and (5) examining the relationship between social competencies and behavior problems and the need for the development of comprehensive, integrated programs to increase the social competence of children with handicaps. These 11 themes provide practitioners and researchers alike with many directions and challenges for the 1990s.

CURRENT PROGRAMS

The early intervention literature on autism is still developing. In some ways it meets the above criteria well, but in some areas virtually no published information is available. This chapter will review several preschool programs for children with autism with Guralnick's (1988) and Karnes and Johnson's (1988) criteria in mind. Although some of these programs have published extensively, most are still in the preliminary stages of evaluating their effectiveness. Thus, a data-based comparison of the projects is not possible. They do, however, illustrate the wide diversity of current data-based approaches to serving preschoolers with autism. We begin with a brief description of 11 widely recognized programs for serving preschool children with autism. We will then discuss the issues raised by Guralnick (1988) and Karnes and Johnson (1988) as they apply to these model programs.

University of California, Los Angeles (UCLA)

Ivar Lovaas' Young Autism Project at UCLA is an ambitious program that provides services to young children with autism in their homes, schools, and communities (Lovaas, 1980, 1987). Through the systematic use of behavioral teaching and some mild aversive techniques (Lovaas, 1981), this program is designed to provide children with intensive programming over almost all their waking hours, 365 days a year. This is accomplished through the use of specially trained student therapists who work in the home and provide training to the child's parents and other caretakers. The UCLA program has received a great deal of media attention since Lovaas' 1987 article reported findings that almost half the children in the experimental group (40 hours of treatment per week for at least 2 years) "recovered from autism" and achieved successful performance in regular first grade classrooms. These data have brought quick criticism from Schopler (1987) and Schopler, Short, and Mesibov (1989), who questioned Lovaas' outcome measures, the adequacy of his control group, and the representativeness of his sample. Lovaas, Smith, and McEachin (1989) have responded to these criticisms and indicated that replication of Lovaas' (1987) study is taking place with improved subject assignment and other methodological changes.

University of Pittsburgh

Since 1982 Phillip Strain and his colleagues at the University of Pittsburgh have operated an integrated preschool known as LEAP (Learning Experiences . . . An Alternative Program for Preschoolers and Parents). Several studies since 1984 have reported on the progress of children with autism and nonhandicapped children using a wide variety of measures. The many components of the program have been specified (Strain, 1987) and include (a) the use of normally developing peers in the teaching of social interaction, (b) individualized group instruction, (c) conceptual and skill training for parents, and (d) transition programming.

Initial reports of outcome (Hoyson, Jamieson, & Strain, 1984; Strain, Hoyson, & Jamieson, 1985; Strain, Jamieson, & Hoyson, 1985) described six "autistic-like" graduates whose scores on the Learning Accomplishment Profile (Sanford & Zelman, 1981) and measures of social interaction increased to normal levels for their ages. By 1988, Strain and Hoyson reported on their follow-up of 26 children, 52% of whom had entered regular education, although some had continued to require smaller classes and more individualized attention than their peers. Of these 26 children, 2 were in classes specifically for children with autism. On a variety of measures, Strain and Hoyson (1988) also indicated better outcome with less program effort for children beginning treatment before 36 months of age. Strain, Jamieson, & Hoyson (1988) reported that the LEAP model has been replicated at 10 other sites.

University of North Carolina at Chapel Hill

Division TEACCH (Treatment and Education of Autistic and related Communication handicapped CHildren) at the University of North Carolina at Chapel Hill has provided services for children and adults with autism and related handicaps since 1971. This statewide program provides both diagnostic and treatment services through its six regional outpatient centers. Operating under the "Parents as Cotherapists" model (Schopler & Reichler, 1971), TEACCH works collaboratively with families and places an emphasis on the development of home teaching programs to help parents work effectively with their handicapped children. In addition, TEACCH provides consultation services to numerous autism classrooms, workshops, and group homes throughout the state (Lansing & Schopler, 1978). Several of the classrooms are designed for preschool children with autism or similar communication handicaps and are typically located in public schools. Preschool children with autism are also served in noncategorical, publicly and privately funded preschool programs or regular preschool or day care programs.

Research has indicated improvements in teaching effectiveness in a sample of 10 mothers (Marcus, Lansing, Andrews, & Schopler, 1978), parent satisfaction (Schopler, Mesibov, & Baker, 1982), and generalization of both child and parent gains from clinic to home settings (Short, 1984). These studies examined TEACCH services over a wide age range. Research on preschool services is in progress.

Princeton Child Development Institute

Fenske, Zalenski, Krantz, and McClannahan (1985) reported on a program that provides "comprehensive behavioral intervention services" for children with autism. The majority of these services are provided in the day school and treatment program at the Princeton

(New Jersey) Child Development Institute. This program employs a behavioral analytic approach to intervention and emphasizes control of problem behavior, development of language skills, and the generalization of skills across people and environments. In addition, children also receive services in the form of individualized parent training conducted in their homes or work in their residential or "transitional settings." Retrospective program evaluation data indicated that children who began intervention earlier (younger than age 5) had more positive outcomes than those who started later (Fenske *et al.*, 1985).

Marshall University

Providing services to families living in rural and isolated areas represents a major challenge. The Preschool Training Project was a federally-funded demonstration program (1985–1988) at Marshall University in Huntington, West Virginia that provided advocacy, training, and consultation services for families in parts of West Virginia, Ohio, and Kentucky (Dunlap, Robbins, Morelli, & Dollman, 1988; Plienis, Robbins, & Dunlap, 1988). Services were provided primarily in the clinic during the initial 3 to 4 month intensive phase of training (approximately 50 to 60 hours of training per child and family) and shifted home and school settings during follow-up (another 50 to 70 hours per training team). Teaching methods were behaviorally based with the emphasis on shaping instructional control during the early parts of training, and training parents and other community care providers during the latter stages of the program.

A total of 15 children and their families participated in the program. All families completed the 3 months of intensive training, and 13 started early enough to complete at least one year. On the average, children made about 10 months of developmental progress over their year of involvement, with some children faring much better than others (Robbins, Dunlap, & Plienis, 1991). During this time, seriously disruptive behavior also decreased (Dunlap, Johnson, & Robbins, 1990).

Delaware Autistic Program

The Delaware Autistic Program is a project of the state's public schools and is located in Newark, Delaware. Preschool services are provided primarily in public school classrooms, with a smaller number (five) of the children in a day care center with project staff support. The preschool program is a part of the larger program serving children and young adults through age 21 (Bondy, 1988, 1989).

The individualized curriculum emphasizes domestic, community, recreation/leisure, communication, behavior management, and some skills commonly needed in regular preschools. The methods are behavioral, and frequent data collection occurs in both one-to-one discrete trial teaching and incidental teaching.

Two special emphases characterize the Delaware program. One is the use of a picture communication system in which children are taught to hand pictures to others to convey a variety of messages. Another is the teaching of alternative behaviors in order to reduce behavior problems.

Transition to first grade is a more straightforward process in Delaware than in most states, because the program is part of the public schools. Program evaluation has involved extensive data showing child progress but no experimental controls or scorer reliability in data collection. The program has been replicated at two other sites in Delaware.

University of Maryland

The University of Maryland Preschool Autism Project (Powers & Egel, 1988, 1989) operates two preschool classes in a regular elementary school in Rockville, Maryland. The 12 autistic children in the program spend parts of each morning in a segregated autism class, and as they acquire specified skills, they are integrated into two Head Start classes located next door. Afternoons are spent in the autism class.

The teaching approach is behavioral with strong emphasis on teaching skills needed for success in Head Start and later environments. This results in a varied curriculum and varied methods, including incidental teaching of language and social skills.

Outcome data for the first two years showed a mean proportional change index above 3.0, indicating a learning rate three times higher than before entering the program. Replication programs have begun at three other sites in the Washington, DC area.

Groden Center

The Kindergarten program of the Groden Center in Providence, Rhode Island provides integrated preschool services in an urban day care center (Stevenson, 1987, 1989). The program has operated since 1984. It places 5 or 6 children with autism and related developmental problems per year in morning day care classes such that one or two of them are integrated with each day care class of about 18 children. In the afternoon the handicapped children attend a segregated program offering intensive instruction.

Instruction is based on behavioral principles and emphasizes social interaction, communication, participation in group activities, play, and self-control of behavior problems. To achieve the latter goal, all children are taught relaxation using methods described by Cautela and Groden (1978). Program evaluation has shown individual child progress but has not used experimental designs.

Rutgers University

Another university-based program is located at Rutgers–The State University in New Brunswick, New Jersey (Harris & Handleman, 1989). The Douglass Developmental Disabilities Center is a day treatment program that provides services for children and young adults from ages 3 to 21, with two classrooms devoted to preschool children. Ten children with autism are served in these two classrooms, with five children integrated with normally developing peers and the other five in a segregated classroom program. The program has a behavioral focus and includes an important parent training component designed to enhance the children's generalization of newly-learned skills. The directors described the Rutgers program as a transitional one, as they prepare the children for their "next environment" by teaching the necessary behaviors to increase the likelihood of success in their next classroom setting.

University of Massachusetts at Amherst

The Walden Learning Center at the University of Massachusetts is an integrated preschool located on the university campus (McGee, 1986, 1988; McGee & Izeman, 1988). The classroom serves seven children with autism and eight nonhandicapped children each year. The children attend for 2 years in a full day, year-round class emphasizing the development of language and social engagement through incidental teaching.

The curriculum stresses social interaction and communication in natural play/learning activities using the normal children as intervention agents. Using incidental teaching, teachers arrange the environment and prompt children to initiate involvement in activities. Although this approach has a behavioral rationale, it stresses child initiation, rather than compliance, and is intended to help foster generalization by bringing behavior under the control of natural cues.

The May Center

Anderson, Avery, DiPietro, Edwards, and Christian (1987) reported on their program in the Boston area, which provides "intensive home-based intervention" for young children with autism. This program represents a partial replication of Lovaas' (1987) model, although it is characterized by services that are less intense and do not include the application of aversive contingencies. Parents are taught skills necessary to manage their children's behavior problems and teach them adaptive behaviors. Staff from the Center spend 15 hours a week in the children's homes and teach parents behavioral teaching strategies and management techniques. The parents commit to providing an additional 10 hours per week of home teaching for their children. Staff also engage in liaison activities with the children's classroom programs. In addition to these family services, the May Center operates several classrooms located in the public schools in the Boston area. Evaluation of the family services yielded child change on several measures and parent gains in the acquisition of teaching skills.

CURRENT ISSUES

The 11 issues raised by Guralnick (1988) and Karnes and Johnson (1988) are well illustrated by programs that offer services to preschool children with autism. These issues may be considered under three headings: curriculum or program issues, measurement, and dissemination.

Curriculum or Program Issues

The following five issues concern characteristics of the preschool programs.

Specifying Program Characteristics

In keeping with their generally behavioral approach, current pre-school programs have been quite explicit in describing what they do. Lovaas' approach is described in a book (Lovaas, 1981), and Strain's curriculum has been made available for replication. Schopler's approach to clinic-based and classroom work with children and their families has been well described (Schopler, Lansing, & Waters, 1983; Schopler, Reichler, & Lansing, 1980) and applied to his preschool services. Although many curricula and program descriptions have not yet been published, clear program description is a strength of current autism programs.

A Clear Educational or Developmental Model

The diversity of models is not as great in current autism preschool programs as it is in programs serving children with other developmental disabilities. Although Schopler's work draws from a developmental and cognitive base (Schopler, Mesibov, Shigley, & Bashford, 1984), the operations of current preschool programs have great similarity in their application of behavioral methods. Within this behavioral framework, programs vary from Lovaas' firm step-by-step approach to McGee's play and exploration format. The common thread is their emphasis on measurement of child behavior and their consistent, systematic application of teaching methods.

Effect of Intensity

"Is more better?" is a reasonable question but a difficult one to answer. Lovaas (1987) is the only researcher in this area to address the question directly by comparing the outcome for two groups. His group receiving more intense services achieved notably better outcome, although the selection of the control group was criticized by Schopler (1987) and Schopler *et al.*, (1989).

Strain's LEAP program has also employed intensive training with dramatic results. However, there are no well controlled comparisons with other, less intensive programs. It can be argued that other programs are less intensive and achieve less child progress, but many factors are confounded with intensity, so conclusions must be guarded.

Anderson *et al.*'s (1987) program was designed to be a less intensive partial replication of Lovaas' model. Their data indicated that none of their children "recovered" from autism. However, their program differed in several key respects from Lovaas' in that their children were somewhat older and perhaps more impaired, and the program did not employ aversive procedures.

Most programs lack the resources or have other limitations that do not allow for the delivery of services as intensive as those of Lovaas. The more practical issue may not be intensive vs. less intensive services but whether the less intensive services that are more feasible will still benefit children. Although outcome data for most of the autism preschool programs cited in this chapter are still preliminary, they have all reported some benefit. As more data become available on current programs, the effect of intensity will become clearer, but for most families the issue is currently some preschool services vs. none.

Social Competencies and Behavior Problems

Children with autism characteristically have deficits in social skills and frequently have behavior problems. Thus, these issues have been central to the provision of preschool services. Lovaas (1987) has been the only recent advocate of even mild punishment to correct behavior problems of preschoolers with autism. Others (Lovaas as well) rely heavily upon teaching social competencies and language as a means of reducing behavior problems.

For many years, an emphasis (some would say overemphasis) has been placed on teaching eye-contact and compliance. More recently a more popular vehicle for teaching social skills has been the placement of preschoolers with autism in classrooms with nonhandicapped peers. In fact, all 11 of the programs described in this chapter have used integration in some way. The best known example is Strain's (e.g., Strain, Hoyson, & Jamieson, 1985) extensive research on peer-mediated instruction. An additional twist on teaching social skills appears in Stevenson's (1987, 1989) program at The Groden Center. Part of her curriculum includes teaching relaxation as a means of self-control. The program uses Cautela and Groden's (1978) methods to substitute socially appropriate (relaxed) behavior for behavior problems.

Thus, these programs appear to be following Guralnick's (1988) suggestions regarding social behavior quite extensively. Although most of the controlled studies have come from Strain, many demonstrations of integration and the teaching of social skills to reduce behavior problems are available.

Broadening Parent Involvement

About 25 years ago the field of autism moved from blaming parents for their children's autism to teaching parents how to help their own children. Today autism services and research have expanded to include an emphasis upon families, their strengths, stresses, and various roles (Powers & Olley, 1989). All of the programs described in this chapter have significant parent components. Schopler has written most extensively about expanding the role of parents (e.g., Schopler et al., 1984).

Some specialized examples of services to families include Anderson et al.'s (1987) program of extensive parent services for children in several preschools. In West Virginia, Dunlap, Robbins, Dollman, and Plienis's (1988) services were primarily for families who then returned to their rural communities to assume diverse roles on behalf of their children.

The current autism programs illustrate well that no single service to families is correct or sufficient. As in other aspects of education, individualization is critical.

Measurement

Often extramural funding is dependent on empirical demonstrations of the effectiveness of early intervention programs. Thus, programs must be prepared to produce data that are not only reliable and valid in the usual sense, but that are meaningful in a much broader sense. The paragraphs to follow will highlight how early intervention programs for children with autism are responding to the measurement issues set forth by Karnes and Johnson (1988) and Guralnick (1988).

Triangulation

Much has been written about the selection of dependent variables and assessment issues for young children with autism and severe handicaps (Casto & Lewis, 1986; Neisworth & Bagnato, 1988; Watson & Marcus, 1988). In their review, Karnes and Johnson (1988) discussed what they termed "triangulation," which refers to the use of multiple dependent measures to gauge program impact. Many of the programs for young children with autism have taken this approach using several different assessment instruments in an attempt to produce convergent data on child outcome (e.g., Anderson *et al.*, 1987; Fenske *et al.*, 1985; Harris & Handleman, 1989; Lovaas, 1987; Plienis *et al.*, 1988; Powers & Egel, 1989). This trend is becoming so pronounced that the use of multiple measures represents more the norm than the exception in the field.

Diversifying Dependent Measures

As Karnes and Johnson (1988) pointed out, the use of multiple measures alone falls short when the goal of assessing the broader impact of programs for young autistic children is considered. These authors concluded that researchers have historically overrelied on IQ tests and have overemphasized child outcome data while excluding information on the program's impact on the family. Although research on preschoolers with autism is still in its early development, several programs have included measures that have assessed how families function (e.g., their coping styles, types of stress they experience) and have used these data to gauge the impact of programs on the family as well as for predictive purposes (e.g., Harris & Handleman, 1989; Plienis *et al.*, 1988; Powers & Egel, 1989).

Describing the Sample and Program

As measurement issues have moved to the forefront in the last few years, almost all the attention has been focused on the specification and selection of dependent variables. Unfortunately, issues related to the description of the independent variables have been relatively neglected. Guralnick (1988), Karnes and Johnson (1988), and Strain (1987) have charged researchers with providing more detailed descriptions of their programs and how the interventions are actually implemented. Closely related to this point is Guralnick's (1988) concern that descriptions of the participants in early intervention programs are usually inadequate. This would seem to be particularly important in autism, as many definitions of this behaviorally defined syndrome are used and generally accepted (American Psychiatric Association, 1980, 1987; National Society for Autistic Children, 1978; Rutter, 1978). By better specifying program and subject information, the field may better understand *what* has worked for *whom*.

When the most recent early intervention programs for autistic children are examined, it is generally the case that the programs *do* specify the criteria used to identify and include children. However, there is a notable lack of consistency across programs. Some employ specified criteria (e.g., American Psychiatric Association, 1980), and others use independent diagnosis by professionals not associated with the program.

Even among children clearly identified as having autism, there is great variability in functioning level and responsiveness to treatment. Therefore, it is important that research and program descriptions indicate IQ levels and the prevalence of other handicaps (e.g., seizure disorders) in their populations. One of Schopler's (1987; Schopler *et al.*, 1989) criticisms of Lovaas' (1987) research was that the UCLA program served disproportionately higher functioning children.

As a practical matter, several of the preschool programs also serve children with handicaps other than autism and older children (e.g., Division TEACCH, Groden Center, Princeton Child Development Institute). Reports of overall program effectiveness do not always break their data down by age and diagnosis; therefore, conclusions are limited. Finally, only a few programs have been described in enough detail that reasonable replication could be expected. Notable in this respect has been the work of Lovaas (1981), Division TEACCH (e.g., Schopler *et al.*, 1980), the Preschool Training Project (Dunlap, Robbins, Dollman, & Plienis, 1988), and LEAP (Strain, Jamieson, & Hoyson, 1985).

Social Validity

A final issue related to measurement discussed by Karnes and Johnson (1988) concerns social validity. Although over 10 years have elapsed since Wolf's (1978) classic paper on social validity, this issue has seldom been raised in autism literature. The work of Schreibman and her colleagues has been a notable exception. They used college undergraduates (Schreibman, Koegel, Mills, & Burke, 1981) and teachers (Schreibman, Runco, Mills, & Koegel, 1982) to validate the effects of parent training with autistic children. Division TEACCH has published data on parent satisfaction (Schopler *et al.*, 1982). Only a few early intervention programs for children with autism have addressed issues related to social validity. For instance, integrated programs have used comparisons with normal children in measuring progress (McGee, 1988; Strain, 1987).

In general, while our ability to define and measure "improvement" in early intervention for children with autism has come far in the last 20 years, many limitations remain. Following the guidelines set forth by Guralnick (1988) and Karnes and Johnson (1988) is an excellent way to start as we seek to improve and refine all aspects of measurement for young children and their families.

Dissemination

It is not enough to develop and implement quality programs for young children with autism. Exemplary programs should emphasize dissemination if the quality of services for all children is to be improved. This is particularly true for areas that have fewer resources and are far removed from the university settings where many leading programs have been developed. Two relevant issues will be discussed in the paragraphs to follow that relate to the general theme of dissemination: replication and impact.

Replication

As Karnes and Johnson (1988) discussed in their review, the concept of replication is often overlooked in early childhood programs. These authors pointed out the importance of replicating research findings across different subjects, settings, behaviors, and methods. Unfortunately, direct replication efforts tend not to be published in scholarly journals, and grant funds are often targeted for innovative programs. Programs for preschoolers with autism also follow this pattern when it comes to replication efforts, although there are two programs that have addressed this important issue. The University of Pittsburgh program (Hoyson *et al.*, 1984; Strain *et al.*, 1985) has been funded to start several "replication classrooms" around the country. Staff from the "home program" in Pittsburgh provide lengthy preservice and in-service training for the staff of the replication programs (Strain *et al.*, 1988). To date, in conjunction with local school systems, several classrooms have been developed nationwide that follow the LEAP curriculum model.

Another program that has been partially replicated has been Ivar Lovaas' Young Autism Project at UCLA. The May Center (Anderson *et al.*, 1987) described their program as a partial replication of the home-based model described by Lovaas. A major difference, however, lies in the intensity of the May Center model, which may, in part, account for the less dramatic results it has achieved (compared with Lovaas, 1987).

Impact

The other area of importance in dissemination concerns the field's ability to expand the impact of its research. Karnes and Johnson (1988) discussed the importance of disseminating research findings to a wider audience than those who read scholarly journals. New approaches must reach practitioners whose efforts can provide significant benefits for the children and families they serve. A second and equally important group that should have access to research findings is policymakers. Detailed research reports filled with jargon and technical language are not likely to receive attention from those who set policy for young children with handicaps. Not surprisingly, the programs for young children with autism described in this chapter suffer from the same shortcomings, with most programmatic research disseminated at professional conferences or in the academic journals. If the burgeoning technologies of the 1980s are to have significant, meaningful, and broad impact, then the 1990s must focus on the wider dissemination of research findings and program descriptions so that practitioners may be able to implement the latest techniques, and policymakers will be able to shape policy (and funding) to benefit all children with handicaps.

ADDITIONAL ISSUES

The issues raised by Guralnick (1988) and Karnes and Johnson (1988) serve to highlight many aspects of current preschool autism services. However, there are additional emphases of the autism programs that have application to all preschool programs. Three such issues are: (a) teaching communication skills; (b) delivering services in a variety of settings; and (c) planning transition from preschool to the next education setting.

Teaching Communication Skills

The importance of communication skills in autism has been addressed extensively elsewhere (e.g., Schopler & Mesibov, 1985; Watson, Lord, Schaffer, & Schopler, 1989), but it is important to point out the key role that communication instruction plays for preschoolers. All 11 programs described in this chapter teach communication skills in a social context. A good example is McGee's (1986, 1988) emphasis upon incidental teaching of language in natural social contexts with nonhandicapped peers. This approach is a departure from individual, discrete trial training, and it has the benefits of social validity and improved generalization of skills. The programs at Rutgers and the Princeton Child Development Institute have also published studies on language teaching for children with autism that have wide application to children with other handicaps. The key feature of the Delaware Autistic Program is its use of a picture communication system both as a language development tool and a potential means to reduce behavior problems (Bondy, 1988).

Service Settings

The autism programs described in this chapter represent a wide variety of settings and formats for services, and they illustrate the ways that services can be adapted to fit local circumstances. For instance, the Massachusetts and Rutgers programs have demonstration preschools on university campuses, and the Princeton Child Development Center is in a private, nonuniversity setting. The UCLA program is a home-and community-based program with later classroom placement. The Groden

Center program is integrated in an urban day care center. The Pittsburgh and North Carolina programs are in regular public schools, and the Maryland program is located in a regular public school with integration in Head Start classes. The Delaware program is operated by the public school system as an extension of their program for older children. The Marshall University program brought families to Huntington, West Virginia, then provided follow-up in local rural communities. Finally, the May Center operates preschool classrooms and provides additional family services for those children as well as children attending other area preschools.

The 11 programs, then, represent a great variety of formats, all of which have demonstrated some success in serving children with autism and their families.

Transition

Regardless of how much progress the children have made in preschool, extensive planning is needed for transition to the next school (Olley & Powers, 1989). Preschool programs serving children with autism have published little on this topic but have demonstrated several approaches. In Delaware, the preschool children move into classes in the same school district operated by the same program. In Maryland, a new kindergarten program was established to provide transition services and avoid placement in a segregated autism classroom.

Although in virtually all programs children are taught the skills they will need to succeed in their next environment, the Maryland and Rutgers programs have taken explicit steps to identify critical skills needed in the next environment and build their curriculum on these skills. In the Maryland preschools, children are integrated into Head Start activities only when they have shown criterion levels of skills in those activities. At Rutgers, children begin transition 6 months before leaving by attending their new classes one day a week with a staff person from the Center.

CONCLUSION

Both research and current practice in early intervention have progressed remarkably in recent years, and services are more readily available to families of children with disabilities then they have ever been. Although the current state of research and practice does not provide the necessary data to determine what approaches are universally best or most effective, this review highlights several important factors.

Can children with autism be identified earlier, and are very early services (e.g., before 36 months) more beneficial? Does more intensive early intervention lead to more child progress? How do individual differences in family systems relate to outcome? How can we better individualize service delivery models to respond to diverse family needs? Under what circumstances does integration with nonhandicapped children benefit children with autism? What format of service delivery is best for local or individual circumstances? What factors promote generalization of gains? What measures best reflect progress? If present trends are good predictors, these questions will be answered in the next decade of research.

REFERENCES

American Psychiatric Association. (1980). *Diagnostic and statistical manual of mental disorders* (3rd ed.). Washington, DC: Author.

American Psychiatric Association. (1987). *Diagnostic and statistical manual of mental disorders* (3rd ed., rev.). Washington, DC: Author.

Anderson, S. R., Avery, D. L., DiPietro, E. K., Edwards, G. L., & Christian, W. P. (1987). Intensive home-based early intervention with autistic children. *Education and Treatment of Children, 10,* 352–366.

Bickman, L., & Weatherford, D. L. (Eds.). (1986). *Evaluating early intervention programs for severely handicapped children and their families.* Austin, TX: Pro-Ed.

Bondy, A. S. (1988, May). *Behavioral research and services for preschool children with autism in Delaware.* Panel discussion at the meeting of the Association for Behavior Analysis, Philadelphia, PA.

Bondy, A. S. (1989, May). *Transition from preschool for children in the Delaware Autistic Program.* Panel discussion at the meeting of the Association for Behavior Analysis, Milwaukee, WI.

Bricker, D., Bailey, E., & Bruder, M. B. (1984). The efficacy of early intervention and the handicapped infant: A wise or wasted resource. In M. Wolraich & D. K. Routh (Eds.), *Advances in developmental and behavioral pediatrics* (Vol. 5, pp. 373–423). Greenwich, CT: JAI Press.

Bryant, D. M., & Ramey, C. T. (1987). An analysis of the effectiveness of early intervention programs for environmentally at-risk children. In M. J. Guralnick & F. C. Bennett (Eds.), *The effectiveness of early intervention for at-risk and handicapped children* (pp. 33–78). Orlando, FL: Academic Press.

Casto, G., & Lewis, A. (1986). Selecting outcome measures in early intervention. *Journal of the Division for Early Childhood, 10,* 118–123.

242   J. GREGORY OLLEY, FRANK R. ROBBINS, and MARLENE MORELLI-ROBBINS

Casto, G., & Mastropieri, M. A. (1986). The efficacy of early intervention programs: A meta-analysis. *Exceptional Children, 52*, 417–424.

Cautela, J. R., & Groden, J. (1978). *Relaxation: A comprehensive manual for adults, children, and children with special needs.* Champaign, IL: Research Press.

Dunlap, G., Johnson, L. F., & Robbins, F. R. (1990). Preventing serious behavior problems through skill development and early intervention. In A. Repp & N. Singh (Eds.) *Perspectives on the use of nonaversive and aversive interventions for persons with developmental disabilities* (pp. 273–286). DeKalb, IL: Sycamore Press.

Dunlap, G., Robbins, F. R., Dollman, C., & Plienis, A. J. (1988). *Early intervention for young children with autism: A regional training approach.* Huntington, WV: Marshall University.

Dunlap, G., Robbins, F. R., Morelli, M. A., & Dollman, C. (1988). Team training for young children with autism: A regional model for service delivery. *Journal of the Division for Early Childhood, 12*, 147–160.

Dunst, C. J., McWilliam, R. A., & Trivette, C. M. (Eds.). (1985). Early intervention. [Special issue]. *Analysis and Intervention in Developmental Disabilities, 5*(1–2).

Dunst, C. J., & Rheingrover, R. M. (1981). An analysis of the efficacy of infant intervention programs with organically handicapped children. *Evaluation and Program Planning, 4*, 287–323.

Farran, D. C. (1990). Effects of intervention with disadvantaged and disabled children: A decade review. In S. J. Meisels & J. Shonkoff (Eds.), *Handbook of early childhood intervention* (pp. 501–539) Cambridge: Cambridge University Press.

Fenske, E. C., Zalenski, S., Krantz, P. J., & McClannahan, L. E. (1985). Age at intervention and treatment outcome for autistic children in a comprehensive intervention program. *Analysis and Intervention in Developmental Disabilities, 5*, 49–58.

Ferry, P. C. (1981). On growing new neurons: Are early intervention programs effective? *Pediatrics, 67*, 38–41.

Fewell, R. R. (Ed.). (1985). Efficacy studies: Programs for young handicapped children [entire issue]. *Topics in Early Childhood Special Education, 5*(2).

Gibson, D., & Fields, D. L. (1984). Early infant stimulation programs for children with Down syndrome: A review of effectiveness. In M. Wolraich & D. K. Routh (Eds.), *Advances in developmental and behavioral pediatrics* (Vol. 5, pp. 331–371). Greenwich, CT: JAI Press.

Guralnick, M. J. (1988). Efficacy research in early childhood intervention programs. In S. L. Odom & M. B. Karnes (Eds.), *Early intervention for infants and children and handicaps: An empirical base* (pp. 75–88). Baltimore: Paul H. Brookes.

Guralnick, M. J., & Bennett, F. C. (Eds.). (1987). *The effectiveness of early intervention for at-risk and handicapped children.* Orlando, FL: Academic Press.

Guralnick, M. J., & Bricker, D. (1987). The effectiveness of early intervention for children with cognitive and general developmental delays. In M. J. Guralnick & F. C. Bennett (Eds.), *The effectiveness of early intervention for at-risk and handicapped children* (pp. 115–173). Orlando, FL: Academic Press.

Harris, S. L., & Handleman, J. S. (1989, May). *Assessing changes in preschool children with autism and their normally developing peers.* Paper presented at the meeting of the Association for Behavior Analysis, Milwaukee, WI.

Hoyson, M., Jamieson, B., & Strain, P. S. (1984). Individualized group instruction of normally developing and autistic-like children: The LEAP curriculum model. *Journal of the Division for Early Childhood, 8*, 157–172.

Karnes, M. B., & Johnson, L. T. (1988). Considerations and future directions for conducting research with young handicapped and at-risk children. In S. L. Odom & M. B. Karnes (Eds.), *Early intervention for infants and children with handicaps: An empirical base* (pp. 287–298). Baltimore: Paul H. Brookes.

Lansing, M., & Schopler, E. (1978). Individualized education: A public school model. In

M. Rutter & E. Schopler (Eds.), *Autism: A reappraisal of concepts and treatment* (pp. 439–452). New York: Plenum Press.

Lovaas, O. I. (1980). Behavioral teaching with young autistic children. In B. Wilcox & A. Thompson (Eds.), *Critical issues in educating autistic children and youth* (pp. 220–233) US Department of Education: Office of Special Education.

Lovaas, O. I. (1981). *Teaching developmentally disabled children: The ME book.* Austin, TX: Pro-Ed.

Lovaas, O. I. (1987). Behavioral treatment and normal educational and intellectual functioning in young autistic children. *Journal of Consulting and Clinical Psychology, 55,* 3–9.

Lovaas, O. I., Smith, T., & McEachin, J. J. (1989). Clarifying comments on the Young Autism Study: Reply to Schopler, Short, and Mesibov. *Journal of Consulting and Clinical Psychology, 57,* 165–167.

Marcus, L. M., Lansing, M., Andrews, C., & Schopler, E. (1978). Improvement of teaching effectiveness in parents of autistic children. *Journal of the American Academy of Child Psychiatry, 17,* 625–639.

McGee, G. G. (1986, May). *Walden Learning Center: An environment for the study and dissemination of incidental teaching technology.* Paper presented at the meeting of the Association for Behavior Analysis, Milwaukee, WI.

McGee, G. G. (1988, July). *The Walden Learning Center.* Paper presented at the meeting of the Autism Society of America, New Orleans, LA.

McGee, G. G., & Izeman, S. (1988, May). *How do kids spend their time in an integrated preschool?* Paper presented at the meeting of the Association for Behavior Analysis, Philadelphia, PA.

Meadow-Orlans, K. (1987). An analysis of the effectiveness of early intervention programs for hearing-impaired children. In M. J. Guralnick & F. C. Bennett (Eds.), *The effectiveness of early intervention for at-risk and handicapped children* (pp. 325–362). Orlando, FL: Academic Press.

National Society for Autistic Children (1978). National Society for Autistic Children definition of the syndrome of autism. *Journal of Autism and Childhood Schizophrenia, 8,* 162–167.

Neisworth, J. T., & Bagnato, S. J. (1988). Assessment in early childhood special education: A typology of dependent measures. In S. L. Odom & M. B. Karnes (Eds.), *Early intervention for infants and children with handicaps: An empirical base* (pp. 23–50). Baltimore: Paul H. Brookes.

Odom, S. L., & Karnes, M. B. (Eds.) (1988). *Early intervention for infants and children with handicaps: An empirical base.* Baltimore: Paul H. Brookes.

Olley, J. G., & Powers, M. D. (Co-chairs). (1989, May). *Transition from preschool to the next environment for children with autism.* Panel discussion at the meeting of the Association for Behavior Analysis, Milwaukee, WI.

Plienis, A. J., Robbins, F. R., & Dunlap, G. (1988). Parent adjustment and family stress as factors in behavioral parent training for young autistic children. *Journal of the Multihandicapped Person, 1,* 31–52.

Powers, M. D., & Egel, A. L. (1988, May). *Child and family factors in preschoolers with autism.* Paper presented at the Association for Behavior Analysis Convention, Philadelphia, PA.

Powers, M. D., & Egel, A. L. (1989, May). *Stress, coping, and conflict in families of young autistic children.* Paper presented at the meeting of the Association for Behavior Analysis, Milwaukee, WI.

Powers, M. D., & Olley, J. G. (Co-chairs). (1989, August). *Research on families of children with autism: Beyond parent training.* Symposium presented at the meeting of the American Psychological Association, New Orleans, LA.

Robbins, F. R., Dunlap, G., & Plienis, A. J. (1991). Family characteristics, family training, and the progress of young children with autism. *Journal of Early Intervention, 15,* 173–184.

Rutter, M. (1978). Diagnosis and definition of childhood autism. *Journal of Autism and Childhood Schizophrenia, 8,* 139–161.

Sanford, A. R., & Zelman, J. G. (1981). *The Learning Accomplishment Profile.* Winston-Salem, NC: Kaplan Press.

Schopler, E. (1987). Lovaas study questioned. *Autism Research Review International, 1*(3), 6.

Schopler, E., Lansing, M., & Waters, L. (1983). *Individualized assessment and treatment for autistic and developmentally disabled children: Vol. 3. Teaching activities for autistic children.* Austin, TX: Pro-Ed.

Schopler, E., & Mesibov, G. B. (Eds.). (1985). *Communication problems in autism.* New York: Plenum Press.

Schopler, E., Mesibov, G. B., & Baker, A. (1982). Evaluation of treatment for autistic children and their parents. *Journal of the American Academy of Child Psychiatry, 21,* 262–267.

Schopler, E., Mesibov, G. B., Shigley, R. H., & Bashford, A. (1984). Helping autistic children through their parents: The TEACCH model. In E. Schopler & G. B. Mesibov (Eds.), *The effects of autism on the family* (pp. 65–81). New York: Plenum Press.

Schopler, E., & Reichler, R. J. (1971). Parents as cotherapists in the treatment of psychotic children. *Journal of Autism and Childhood Schizophrenia, 1,* 87–102.

Schopler, E., Reichler, R. J., & Lansing, M. (1980). *Individualized assessment and treatment for autistic and developmentally disabled children: Vol. 2. Teaching strategies for parents and professionals.* Austin, TX: Pro-Ed.

Schopler, E., Short, A., & Mesibov, G. (1989). Relation of behavioral treatment to "normal functioning": Comment on Lovaas. *Journal of Consulting and Clinical Psychology, 57,* 162–164.

Schreibman, L., Koegel, R. L., Mills, J. I., & Burke, J. C. (1981). Social validation of behavior therapy with autistic children. *Behavior Therapy, 12,* 610–624.

Schreibman, L., Runco, M. A., Mills, J. I., & Koegel, R. L. (1982). Teachers' judgements of improvements in autistic children in behavior therapy: A social validation. In R. L. Koegel, A. Rincover, & A. L. Egel (Eds.), *Educating and understanding autistic children* (pp. 78–87). San Diego: College-Hill Press.

Short, A. B. (1984). Short-term treatment outcome using parents as cotherapists for their own autistic children. *Journal of Child Psychology and Psychiatry and Allied Disciplines, 25,* 443–458.

Simeonsson, R. J., Cooper, D. H., & Schiener, A. P. (1982). A review and analysis of the effectiveness of early intervention programs, *Pediatrics, 69,* 635–641.

Simeonsson, R. J., Olley, J. G., & Rosenthal, S. L. (1987). Early intervention for children with autism. In M. J. Guralnick & F. C. Bennett (Eds.), *The effectiveness of early intervention for at-risk and handicapped children* (pp. 275–296). Orlando, FL: Academic Press.

Stevenson, S. E. (1987). *Forming cooperative programs for mainstreaming preschool children with severe behavior disorders: Policy, programmatic, and procedural issues.* Providence, RI: The Groden Center. (ERIC Document Reproduction Service No. ED 294–354).

Stevenson, S. E. (1989, July). *Critical elements in the establishment and operation of educational settings for preschool children with autism.* Paper presented at the meeting of the Autism Society of America, Seattle, WA.

Strain, P. S. (1987). Comprehensive evaluation of intervention for young autistic children. *Topics in Early Childhood Special Education, 7*(2), 97–110.

Strain, P. S., & Hoyson, M. (1988, July). *Follow-up of children in LEAP.* Paper presented at the meeting of the Autism Society of America, New Orleans, LA.

Strain, P. S., Hoyson, M. H., & Jamieson, B. J. (1985). Normally developing preschoolers as intervention agents for autistic-like children: Effects on class deportment and social interactions. *Journal of the Division for Early Childhood, 9,* 105–115.

Strain, P. S., Jamieson, B. J., & Hoyson, M. H. (1985). Learning Experiences. An Alternative Program for Preschoolers and Parents: A comprehensive service system for the mainstreaming of autistic-like preschoolers. In C. J. Meisel (Ed.), *Mainstreamed handicapped children: Outcomes, controversies, and new directions* (pp. 251–269). Hillsdale, NJ: Erlbaum.

Strain, P. S., Jamieson, B. J., & Hoyson, M. H. (1988, May). *Replication of the LEAP model program for young autistic children.* Paper presented at the meeting of the Association for Behavior Analysis, Philadelphia, PA.

Watson, L. R., Lord, C., Schaffer, B., & Schopler, E. (1989). *Teaching spontaneous communication to autistic and developmentally handicapped children.* Austin, TX: Pro-Ed.

Watson, L. R., & Marcus, L. M. (1988). Diagnosis and assessment of preschool children. In E. Schopler & G. B. Mesibov (Eds.), *Diagnosis and assessment in autism* (pp. 271–302). New York: Plenum Press.

White, K. R., & Casto, G. (1984). An integrative review of early intervention efficacy studies with at-risk children: Implications for the handicapped. *Analysis and Intervention in Developmental Disabilities, 5,* 7–31.

Wolf, M. M. (1978). Social validity: The case for subjective measurement or how applied behavior analysis is finding its heart. *Journal of Applied Behavior Analysis, 11,* 203–214.

12

Federal Legislation for
Young Children with Disabilities

JUDITH E. THIELE

INTRODUCTION

Other chapters in this volume have addressed issues of identification
and treatment of infants or young children with autism or related disabilities. This chapter describes key features of the federal legislation,
Individuals with Disabilities Education Act (IDEA), that has provided
much of the impetus for changes in policies and funding for services
for these young children. The chapter describes the context in which
the legislation was passed and outlines key features of a "free and
appropriate public education" which is guaranteed to those aged 3 to 21
and services extended to children from birth through age 2 and their
families under the legislation. This description will address services to
be provided to individual children aged 3 to 5 and from birth through
age 2, rights guaranteed to parents and children in accessing those
services, and requirements that states must meet in order to qualify for
the federal funding, including an overview of parents' rights in reviewing and approving state plans.

Because few states provide compulsory education for preschool
children, legislation mandates for placement of preschool children with

JUDITH E. THIELE • Children's Rehabilitation Unit, University of Kansas Medical Center, Kansas City, Kansas 66160-7340.

Preschool Issues in Autism, edited by Eric Schopler *et al.* Plenum Press, New York, 1993.

disabilities in the least restrictive, appropriate settings raise special challenges for educators. For this reason, the concepts of least restrictive
environment and interagency cooperation are discussed in some detail.
Special provisions of the law that apply to infants and toddlers are then
discussed, followed by a brief discussion of additional, related research
and service programs authorized under the same legislation.

The IDEA Amendments of 1991 (Public Law 102-119) authorized Federal assistance to states to provide early intervention for children with disabilities. Two programs are included to provide services
for preschool children and infants, toddlers, and their families. The
Preschool Grants Program (Part B) provides assistance to states for
special education and related services for preschool children aged 3
through 5 with disabilities; and the Handicapped Infant and Toddler
Program (Part H) provides assistance to states to develop a comprehensive system of early intervention for infants and toddlers from birth
through 2 years and their families. At a time when Congress enacted
legislation to balance the Federal budget (Omnibus Budget Reconciliation Act, known as Gramm, Rudman, & Hollings, 1981), and many
social support programs received drastic budget cuts, a major commitment was made to our youngest and most vulnerable children. Until the
1980's, Federal support for early intervention was limited to the Head
Start Program and the Handicapped Children's Early Education Program. Although these programs were designed to develop or improve
early educational opportunities for children under 5 years, the services
have not been available to all eligible children.

In 1986, the Education of the Handicapped Act (EHA) Public Law
99-457 sharply increased assistance to states to provide children aged 3
through 5 years a free appropriate public education (FAPE). This program
was the principal source of federal aid to state and local school systems
for instructional and support services for preschool children with disabilities. In 1991, the EHA was reauthorized by Congress and renamed Individuals with Disabilities Education Act (IDEA), Public Law 102-119.

A NEW AGE IN EARLY INTERVENTION
AND PRESCHOOL EDUCATION

IDEA, Public Law 102-119, is one of the most far-reaching federal
laws to touch the lives of young children with disabilities and their

families. The centerpiece of the Act is a state grant-in-aid program, authorized under Part B, which includes the current Preschool Grants Program for children aged 3 through 5 years. Overall Federal funding for the Preschool Grants Program during Fiscal Year 1992 was $175 million, which was a 50% increase over the previous year, and 3½ times the amount ($50 million) authorized in 1987.

Although initially IDEA (Public Law 94-142, passed in 1975), for children aged 5 through 17 years, was authorized to provide funding equal to 40% of the cost (determined by the national average per pupil expenditure times the nation's special education child count), the Federal share has never exceeded 12% (National Council on Disability, 1989). The Federal share of support for special education and related services for preschool children with disabilities is now about 6% of the national average cost to state and local agencies, less than one-fourth of what could be authorized. In spite of the small Federal contribution, it is remarkable that so much has been accomplished under IDEA and that opportunities for preschool children who need special education continue to expand.

THE PRESCHOOL GRANTS PROGRAM

Free and Appropriate Public Education

The Basic State Grants for the Education of Children with Disabilities (Part B) requires participating states to furnish all children and young adults aged 3 through 21 years with disabilities with FAPE, in the least restrictive setting by school year 1991–92. The purpose of the Part B formula grants is to assist states in covering part of the cost of providing special education and related services to handicapped children, under the provisions of FAPE and in the least restrictive setting. A "free appropriate public education" includes:

1. Special education, defined as "specially designed instruction to meet the unique needs of a child with disabilities, including classroom instruction, instruction in physical education, home instruction and instruction in hospitals and institutions"; and
2. Related services, defined as: "transportation, and such developmental, corrective and other supportive services . . . as may

be required to assist a child with disabilities to benefit from special education . . . ," including speech pathology and audiology, psychological services, physical and occupational therapy, recreation, medical and counseling services (for evaluation purposes), and early identification and assessment of disabilities in children.

Special education and related services are to be provided at no cost to parents, and as a part of an individualized education program (IEP) developed with parent collaboration and consent for each preschool child age 3 through 5 by school year 1991–92. The same parental rights that assure the provision of FAPE to school-age students with disabilities also apply to preschool children with special needs:

1. A *zero reject* policy that assures all children with disabilities the right to a free appropriate public education;
2. An *individualized education program* for each child with a disability is required of the local educational agency;
3. Established *due process,* or the right of parents to question or challenge plans by the school prior to any action that will affect their child's education;
4. Procedures for *integrating handicapped students into the least restrictive setting* such as the regular classroom to the maximum extent appropriate;
5. *Nondiscriminatory testing and evaluation* that is racially and culturally unbiased.

State Level Provisions

Four additional provisions of EHA-Part B are important elements of building a "comprehensive delivery system" of special education for preschool children:

1. A *state plan,* policies, and procedures for providing special education and related services that conforms to the definitions in the Act;
2. Establishes *the needs of unserved children with disabilities* as top priority and second priority to improving services to underserved children with the most severe disabilities;
3. *Assignment to the state educational agency* the responsibility

for carrying out the provisions of program, including general supervision of special education administered by state or local agencies.

4. *Shared decision making* with concerned persons and parents through public hearings to obtain input prior to adopting policies, programs, and procedures.

All of these elements are required under IDEA-Part B and are the mechanisms through which the development or expansion of special education and related services for preschool children in each state can be affected. Teachers and parents can examine a state plan to: determine the level of Federal and state support contributed to preschool children; determine the extent to which unserved or underserved preschool children with disabilities are a top priority in their state; identify who in their assigned state educational agency is responsible for preschool special education and related services; and participate in shared decisionmaking to form policies and develop programs and procedures for preschool youngsters with disabilities.

Until 1991, under section 619(b)(1) of IDEA-Part B, a state had to qualify for basic Part B funding, have an approved early childhood education plan and serve some, but not necessarily all, youngsters with disabilities between 3 and 5 years of age. Since 1991, the Secretary of Education may award grants only to states which: (1) meet the eligibility requirements for Part B grants (i.e., basic grants to the states for educating handicapped children aged 3 through 21 years of age); and (b) have an approved state plan that assures the availability under state law and practice of a free, appropriate public education for all handicapped children aged 3 through 5 years.

These basic provisions are the foundation of the Preschool Grants Program authorized under this federal legislation. Separate allotments are made to states under Part B to encourage the provision of special education and related services to preschool children aged 3 through 5 with disabilities. The 1986 Amendments to IDEA brought many changes, including three separate programs for preschool children, infants and toddlers, and school-age children. The law emphasizes interagency coordination of services and gives a great deal of latitude to states to assign responsibility and to establish new policies for early intervention and preschool services (Fowler *et al.,* 1990; Rice & O'Brien, 1990). Although many states are revising policies to create specific identification, assessment and placement procedures for preschool children, issues such as transition between programs, eligibility criteria, implementation strategies, and personnel standards are challenges to all the states.

Failure to Comply

All states must assure the provision of FAPE to all eligible preschoolers or risk the sanctions provided in the federal statute. These sanctions include the loss of: Part B preschool funds; Part B state grant funds for children 3 to 5 years of age; Chapter I handicapped funds for children 3 to 5 years old; and discretionary funds under IDEA, Parts C–G, relating to preschool special education services.

Special Issues in Serving Young Children

State participation in the Preschool Grants Program raises a number of issues for administrators, teachers, parents and other service providers. Existing policies and regulations that assure the provision of FAPE and a continuum of Least Restrictive Environments (LRE) may not result in appropriate practices for preschool children with disabilities. Assessment procedures, personnel qualifications, and transition practices have been designed to meet the needs of school age children and may not be appropriate for preschool children with disabilities.

Establishing the policies and criteria for the Preschool Grants Program is proving to be a challenge to most states. In a survey of states and territories (Walsh & McKenna, 1988) 49 of the 57 states and territories responded to questions about changes in least restrictive environment, transition practices, and interagency agreements to implement the Preschool Grants Program.

Least Restrictive Environment

By 1990, one fourth of the states had developed LRE policies or guidelines specific for preschool programs to assure that all children aged 3 through 5 years with disabilities received a FAPE in the least restrictive environment. Ten other states were in the process of developing LRE policies specifically for preschool children, and in the remaining states, the IDEA-B policies for all special education programs were applied to preschool children. Providing a continuum of placement options that are flexible and meet the unique needs of children and young adults throughout the age range of birth through 21 continues to be a challenge to all states. Such policies for preschool children must support the development of education settings that include age peers without disabilities, flexible placement options that provide transportation, and transition support services.

Many state agency personnel raise concerns about providing preschool services in each child's LRE. For example, educational settings that include preschoolers without disabilities are not widely available to, or under the supervision of, administering educational agencies. Preschoolers in need of speech and language therapy may not have the opportunity to interact with peers who do not need such therapy. The least restrictive educational setting for these youngsters are programs that can offer opportunities to interact with their age peers, who can provide appropriate language models. Although a few model LRE projects exist and are successful, many school districts have started segregated preschools (McKenna, 1989).

Interagency Coordination

Interagency agreements between State Educational Agencies (SEA) and other agencies can provide placement options to the SEA that include settings to establish integrated preschools. The array of preschool services needed to assure a continuum of LRE for preschoolers with disabilities (transportation, settings for preschoolers without disabilities, personnel standards) make agreements between the SEAs and Head Start, Developmental Disabilities, and the Departments of Health, Human, and Social Services an important outcome of interagency coordination.

Over half of the SEAs have developed interagency agreements with Head Start programs to provide less restrictive placements for many preschoolers with disabilities. Although the standards for personnel qualifications in the Head Start Program do not match the personnel standards under the supervision of SEAs, many states have developed agreements with Head Start programs to meet the more stringent personnel standards of IDEA. Interagency agreements between Head Start and the SEA range from shared classrooms (under general supervision of the Educational Agency) for both programs, to Itinerate Teacher staffing models for the IDEA preschoolers in Head Start classrooms (provides a certified teacher to supervise the Individualized Education Plans for each preschooler receiving FAPE). These arrangements provide less restrictive placement options for many preschoolers and they meet the IDEA standards of personnel qualifications.

Transition Services

Smooth transition into the preschool program and into programs for children aged 5 to 21 years is often difficult for the child, family, and many of the professionals involved. The reauthorization of IDEA included several changes to the preschool (Part B) and infant and toddler (Part H) programs designed to develop a "seamless" system of services for children from birth to age 5, and their families. These changes are expected to ensure a smooth transition for children moving from early intervention programs under Part H to preschool programs under part B and to ensure the delivery of appropriate services.

Under the reauthorization, state policies and procedures are required that include a definition of how the state will ensure a smooth transition at age 3 and a description of how parents will be included in transition planning. At least 90 days before the child is eligible for preschool services, a conference between the preschool and early intervention program personnel and the family must be convened to review the child's program options from the third birthday through the rest of the school year and to establish a plan for transition activities (e.g., visits to the new program for the child and family, conferences between the teachers of both programs, etc.).

Prior to the reauthorization of IDEA, money was allocated separately to the infant and toddler program and to the preschool program. Now, states can use Part H funds to pay for children who turn 3 during the school year and up to 20% of preschool grant funds may be used to pay for children who will turn 3 during the school year (whether or not these children have received Part H services).

The Individualized Family Service Plan (IFSP), the equivalent to the preschool program's Individualized Education Plan (IEP), can now be used for a child making the transition into a preschool program, with a parent's permission. The IFSP can be used throughout the child's tenure in a preschool program or until the child is 5 years old, if parents agree.

The changes made by Congress to erase the dividing lines between the infant and toddler, and preschool programs was driven by the notion of a "seamless" program of services for children from birth through 5 years and their families, in order to promote smooth transition between programs and to ensure that comprehensive, appropriate services are delivered.

INFANT AND TODDLER PROGRAM (PART H)

Although this book focuses on the preschool years, Part H is inextricably related to the future of comprehensive and continuous services for all young children with disabilities and their families. In this section, the major components of Part H are described and related programs are discussed. This federal program is designed to assist States in establishing a comprehensive, statewide system of early intervention services that meets the unique needs of infants and toddlers with disabilities and their families. Regulations for infants and toddlers (birth through 2 years) served under this legislation (Federal Register, 34 CFR Part 303, 1989) are similar in many respects to those for the Preschool Grants Program for children aged 3 through 5. The regulations include incentives to assure that all infants and toddlers with disabilities receive certain essential services; a guarantee of due process procedures to assure parents' rights to question or challenge plans made for their child, and to safeguard the confidentiality of information regarding their child; requirements for appropriate evaluation procedures by qualified personnel; placement in the least restrictive environment; a strong focus on interagency coordination of care; collaboration with parents in designing and monitoring the child's intervention program; and provisions for a smooth transition into the preschool program for eligible children.

Specific features of the infant/toddler program, however, reflect special problems in diagnosing very young children and respond to the range of service needs, service settings (e.g., homes, hospitals, day care, etc.), and varied funding sources appropriate for infants and toddlers (Thiele & Hamilton, 1991). Infants and toddlers with developmental delays in one or more functional areas are eligible for services as are children with diagnosed medical or physical conditions that are likely to result in developmental delay (e.g., children with Down Syndrome or sensory impairments). At their discretion, states can also choose to define and include infants and toddlers "at risk of having substantial developmental delays if early intervention services were not provided" (Federal Register, 34 CFR 303.16 (2) b, p. 26313).

One of the most significant features of this legislation is the mandate for an Individualized Family Service Plan (IFSP). For each child, a plan is developed jointly by the family and early intervention personnel. Based on a multidisciplinary evaluation of the child and the child's family, the IFSP includes services that, with the parent's consent, will enhance the development of the child and the capacity of the family to meet the special needs of the child. This plan includes information about the current status of the child, a statement of the family's expressed resources and needs if desired by the family, outcomes to be achieved for the child and the family, the specific services necessary to meet the needs of the child and family, and procedures for transition into preschool education for eligible children. (For a detailed discussion of issues related to the IFSP, see Fewell, 1991).

Unlike services for preschool children (aged 3 through 5), not all intervention and related services must be provided free of charge unless currently required under state law. No fees may be charged for child find procedures that identify potentially eligible children, for required evaluations and assessments, for services coordination, or for administrative and coordinating activities related to the Individualized Family Service Plan (IFSP) or implementation of due process safeguards. A sliding fee schedule can be used for services that the child is not otherwise entitled to without charge, and provision is made to guarantee services for parents unable to pay.

To ensure coordination across existing state agencies and funding sources, the legislation provides for state interagency agreements that define the clinical and fiscal responsibilities of participating agencies, the creation of a State Interagency Coordination Council (ICC) to assist the lead agency in coordination and implementation, and regulations to prevent supplanting of existing services or funding sources with these federal monies. ICC membership must include the representative heads of service agencies, service providers, and parents of children with disabilities from birth through 8 years of age.

OTHER PROGRAMS

In addition to Part B and Part H of IDEA, programs for demonstration, experimental, outreach, research, training, and technical assistance projects are authorized under Part C of IDEA. The Early Education for Children with Disabilities Program (EECDP) (formerly the Handicapped Children's Early Education Program, HCEEP) supports projects which focus on services to children with disabilities from birth through age 8 years, with an emphasis on children under age six. Parent participation, dissemination of information to professionals and the general public, and evaluation of the effectiveness of each project are required. This program is intended to improve the quality of early education and intervention by funding research and development projects of a limited duration which are awarded to state, local, university, and private organizations. EECDP funds approximately 120 projects annually to develop and evaluate educational or developmental strategies for young children with disabilities and their families.

The discretionary programs under IDEA are another source of Federal funds available to State and Local Educational Agencies, and other public, private, for-profit and not-for-profit agencies. These programs serve as a support system to the State grant programs. Funds are available to initiate, expand, and improve special education and early intervention services for children who are below school age. With the passage of IDEA, Public Law 102-119, Congress significantly strengthened discretionary support for the purpose of increasing states' capacity to meet the needs of young children with disabilities as well as those at risk of developmental delay.

The Early Education for Children with Disabilities Program is the single largest source of discretionary funds supporting initiatives in the areas discussed above. Comprised of multiple program components, this program funds demonstrations, outreach projects, experimental projects, technical assistance, research institutes, and inservice personnel development activities.

Services for deaf-blind children and youth are included in a separate program authorized under Part C of IDEA. The Secretary of Education is authorized to award grants or enter into cooperative agreements or contracts with public or nonprofit private agencies, institutions, or organizations to assist SEAs in educating deaf-blind children and youth and helping them to make a successful transition from school to adult life. The grantee/contractor is responsible for providing technical assistance, preservice and inservice training, replication of innovative approaches, and facilitating parental involvement. Grants, cooperative agreements, and contracts are also authorized to support regional technical assistance programs and for the development of extended school year demonstration programs for children and youth with severe disabilities, including deaf-blind children and youth.

Other programs that provide special education to preschool children include Chapter I of the Education Consolidation and Improvement Act of 1981, which includes special education for children with disabilities and migrant children, under age 21 and economically disadvantaged. Approximately 12% of all Head Start enrollees are children with disabilities, and whose families are economically disadvantaged.

SUMMARY: COMPREHENSIVE SERVICE DELIVERY

The delivery of special services to preschool children involves the coordination of a wide range of services provided by multiple public and private agencies at the state and local level. For several reasons, service delivery is substantially different for very young children than for their school age peers. For example, the public school serves as the logical focal point for the development and delivery of services to school age children with disabilities, and, in some states, for younger children. However, in most states, no such single agency or point of contact is designated at the local level to oversee the provision of free, appropriate special education for preschoolers with disabilities.

Because of the age of these young children, service delivery designed to meet their needs must also take into consideration the needs and role of child/daycare providers and the family as primary caregivers. Appropriate service sites for children in this age group are considerably more diverse than for older children, and include the home, day care centers, hospitals and clinics, and private and publicly supported preschool programs. Further complicating the delivery of services is the fact that the needs of very young children with disabilities are often complex, involving medical, psychological, and developmental problems. Services to meet these needs are typically provided by different agencies and under differing authorities. Generally, these agencies maintain their own policies regarding such matters as eligibility for the services they provide, financing of such services, and the personnel qualified or required to provide the services. Finally, while the need to provide early education and related services has been widely acknowledged for many years, only a handful of states require that comprehensive services be provided to all children under age 3 with disabilities.

AUTHOR'S NOTE

Preparation of this manuscript was completed while serving as an Education Research Analyst in the Early Childhood Branch of the Office of Special Education Programs, U.S. Department of Education. However, since the opinions expressed herein do not necessarily reflect the position or policy of the U.S. Department of Education, no official endorsement by the department should be inferred.

ACKNOWLEDGMENT

The Author would like to thank Drs. James L. Hamilton, Susan A. Fowler, and Marie M. Bristol for their helpful comments and suggestions on the preparation of this chapter.

REFERENCES

Education of the Handicapped Act, P.L. 99-457, 20 U.S.C. 1471-1485, C.F.D.A.: 84.181.
Federal Register, Part III, Department of Education, 34 CFR Part 303, p. 17, June 22, 1989.
Fewell, R. (Ed.). (1991). Individualized Family Service Plans. [Special Issue]. *Topics in Early Childhood Special Education, 11*(3), 54–65.
Fowler, S. A., Hains, A. H., & Rosenkoetter, S. E. (1990). The transition between early intervention services and preschool services: Administration and policy issues. *Topics in Early Childhood Special Education, 9*(4), 55–65.
McKenna, P. (1989). Survey of states and territories concerning changes in state authorities to implement the preschool grants program. *National Association of State Directors of Special Education, Inc.* Washington, DC
Omnibus Budget Reconciliation Act, P.L. 97-35, 1981.

Part B, Education of the Handicapped Act as amended by P.L. 94-142, P.L. 98-199, P.L. 99-457 and others. 20 U.S.C. 1419, C.F.D.A.: 84.173.

Part C, Education of the Handicapped Act (P.L. 91-230), as amended by 99-457. 20 U.S.C. 1423. C.F.D.A.: 84.024.

Part H, Education of the Handicapped Act, as amended by P.L. 99-457. 20 U.S.C. 1471-1485. C.F.D.A.: 84.181.

Rice, M. L., & O'Brien, M. (1990). Transitions: Times of change and accommodation. *Topics in Early Childhood Special Education, 9*(4), 1–14.

Subcommittee on the Handicapped, *Report on Education of the Handicapped Act,* as amended through December 31, 1975. Washington, DC: U.S. Government Printing Office. August 1976, 26.

Thiele, J. E., & Hamilton, J. L. (1991). Implementing the early childhood formula: Programs under P.L. 99-457. *Journal of Early Intervention, 15*(1), 5–12.

Walsh, S., & McKenna, P. (1988). A survey of states and territories concerning changes in authorities to implement the preschool grants program. *National Association of State Directors of Special Education, Inc.* Washington, DC

Author Index

Subject Index